1,001 PEARLS OF
YOGA WISDOM

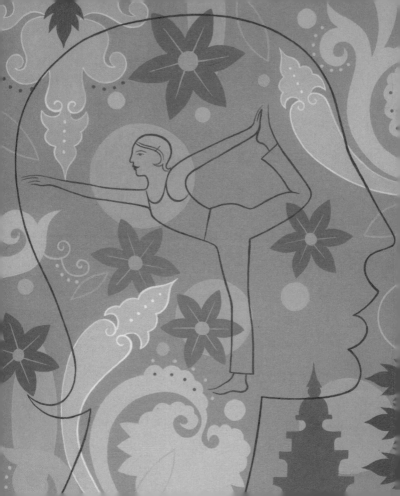

1,001 PEARLS OF YOGA WISDOM

Take Your Practice Beyond the Mat   Liz Lark

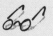

CHRONICLE BOOKS

San Francisco

1001 Pearls of Yoga Wisdom
Liz Lark

First published in the United States
in 2008 by Chronicle Books LLC.

First published in the United Kingdom and
Ireland in 2008 by Duncan Baird Publishers.

Library of Congress Cataloging-in-Publication Data
available.
ISBN: 978-0-8118-6358-2
Manufactured in Thailand

Conceived, created, and designed by Duncan Baird
Publishers.

Managing Editor: Kelly Thompson
Editor: Susannah Marriott
Editorial Assistants: Emma Maule, Kirty Topiwala
Managing Designer: Daniel Sturges
Commissioned Artwork: Tracy Walker / i2i Art

Typeset in AT Shannon

10 9 8 7 6 5 4 3 2

Chronicle Books LLC
680 Second Street
San Francisco, California 94107

www.chroniclebooks.com

Publisher's note: The information in this book
is not intended as a substitute for professional
medical advice and treatment. If you are pregnant
or suffering from any health problems, consult
a medical professional before following any of
the advice suggested in this book. Duncan Baird
Publishers, or any other persons involved in creating
this publication, cannot accept responsibility for any
injuries or damage incurred as a result of following
the information or exercises contained in this book.

➤ This symbol denotes a yoga posture, and
is always followed by the pearl number
of the next posture in the book.

CONTENTS

INTRODUCTION

Yoga is all about relationships – your relationship with yourself, with the people in your life and with the world around you. This makes the yoga path a journey of connection – both internal and external. Indeed, the Sanskrit root from which the word *yoga* derives – *yuj* – means "to yoke", or to connect. In this book, I offer you 1001 ways to "connect".

Many people think of yoga as either a system of physical exercise or a calming means of escapism from the chaotic world. Yoga can be either of these but it is also much more: I see it as a way of exploring both the body and the mind, and through such enquiry, of realizing and "connecting with" our vast untapped potential. Yoga – both on and off the mat – offers each and every one of us a metaphorical ladder – toward *jivanmukti*, liberation in life. As we climb the rungs of this ladder, we take on the yoga viewpoint, or *dharshana*, and ascend out of a world of stress, worry and limitations. We can learn to see beyond ourselves and develop the relationship with our higher, more contented "self".

Yoga works with the raw material common to each of us no matter where or how we live – our bodies, breath, mind and emotions. You might like to think of this raw material as pebbles picked up from a beach, which you can hone and polish until they eventually become precious stones. There are no gadgets in which to refine the stones to perfection. Instead, yoga simply urges us to use what we've got – to take the time to look inside ourselves and find ways of reconnecting with who we really are – uncovering our unpolished but beautiful inner "pebbles", which we all too often lose sight of in today's fast-moving, achievement-driven society. So, the next time life feels rife with mental stress and physical tension, yoga can help you to find ways to ride, and even transcend, this "sea of sorrows". A regular spiritual, mental and physical yoga practice can empower and ground you, helping you to bring stress under control and to cultivate balance and life-purpose amid the chaos.

The 1001 pearls that follow present yoga in its broadest sense (philosophy and practice) and aspire to remove yogic concepts such as asanas, mantras, pranayama and meditation from the esoteric pedestals on which they often sit in people's minds, making them just as accessible and beneficial to beginners as they are inspirational and valuable to more experienced yoga practitioners. May the words in these pearls kickstart not only your physical and mental well-being but also your spiritual connections, taking you on a journey inward, toward the heart, and also outward, to connect with the entire universe.

The yoga path perceives that heaven lies within us. I hope that this book inspires you to explore this rewarding and heavenly path. Namaste!

PEARLS OF WISDOM

There are as many hidden chinks of wisdom in yoga as there are points of
light in a diamond, and the pages that follow aim to draw your attention
to a selection of the most significant "points of light", or yogic teachings.
The 1001 "pearls" not only present wise words from ancient Hindu
texts for you to mull over and inspiring thoughts from contemporary
swamis and gurus for you to take on board. They also offer a grounding
in fundamental yoga concepts, fascinating explanations of many yogic
terms, insight into the body's subtle energy system, translations of key

Sanskrit words, enchanting tales from Hindu mythology and religion, and, of course, a wealth of practical information – whether in the form of guidance on asanas (yoga postures), mantras (sacred sounds), mudras (hand, body or eye gestures), pranayama (breathing techniques), meditations, visualizations or *bandhas* (subtle energy locks).

The aim is quite simple: to encourage you to integrate yoga, in all its forms, into your everyday life – to "live" yoga no less! Note to self: you can benefit from yoga's numerous health-enhancing properties without (necessarily!) retreating to a mountain top or renouncing worldly living. In fact, you don't even have to do asanas to practise; you can do yoga while lying in bed, taking a shower, walking down the street or indeed reading this book. This is because, ultimately, it's about finding a certain quality of attention and awareness, which will enhance your well-being and enrich every part of your daily experience.

The pearls of wisdom that follow are presented in chapters that broadly follow the cycle of a day – from getting up and going to work to coming home in the evening and winding down before bed. That way, you can dip into whichever chapter feels most relevant to your needs at any given time. I hope this treasure trove of yogic insight will help you to live a happier, less stressful, more fulfilling life.

THE ORIGINS OF YOGA

It is useful to know a little about the roots of yoga before setting out on your own yoga journey. We have no way of knowing for sure how long people have been practising the yogic way of life, but it's believed that this wisdom was passed down orally from guru to disciple during ancient India's Vedic Age – as a means of living a harmonious and spiritually connected life. The word *vedic* derives from the Sanskrit root *vid*, meaning knowledge, and the writings of this age – known as the *Vedas*, which consist of four books and convey key Hindu teachings – contain the earliest known written records of yoga. Other yogic texts followed throughout the ages (see right for key titles), and inspirational quotes from many of these appear throughout this book.

Although yoga is now widely practised across the globe, it was only in the 1960s that it first captured the attention and imagination of people in the West due to an influx of Indian teachers. Since then, it has grown enormously in popularity; a key figure in this growth being Swami Sivananda, who established The Five Pillars of yoga practice (see p23).

KEY YOGA TEXTS

• **Upanishads** Originally transmitted orally, this follow-on to the four main Vedic texts (see left) is thought to have first been written down around 800 BCE. Describing an ancient way of living appropriate to higher-caste Hindu men and renunciates, based mainly on study, contemplation and meditation, this text is now an inspiration to anyone interested in pursuing a yogic way of life.

• **Bhagavad Gita** Forming the kernel at the heart of the epic Indian story the *Mahabharata*, the *Gita* is thought to have been written around 400–300 BCE (by anonymous sages). It describes a symbolic spiritual battle, as its narrator, Lord Krishna, explains to the warrior Arjuna valuable tenets of yoga philosophy to follow: mainly the ways of wisdom (*jnana*), devotion (*bhakti*) and selfless action (*karma*).

• **Yoga Sutras** The Sanskrit word *sutra* means "thread" – in this case a string of 185 aphorisms or "wisdoms" about the yogic lifestyle. These are the teachings of the most recognized sage of hatha yoga, Patanjali, who is thought to have lived in the 2nd or 3rd centuries CE. Although written some 2,000 years ago, this text sets out the eight-limbed path of yoga that many still observe today (see pp14–15).

• **Hatha Yoga Pradipika** Written by the sage Swatmarama Yogindra in the mid-14th century, this is considered to be the earliest written instruction manual purely on hatha yoga and it remains the primary text on the subject today, with descriptions of postures (asanas), breathing practices (pranayama), gestures (mudras), cleansing techniques (*kriyas*) and energy locks (*bandhas*).

YOGA PATHS

All yoga leads to the same conclusion – a connection with the divine,
or your "true", transcendent self, and thus a sense of inner wholeness.
However, we can choose to travel along a number of different paths to
reach this point, depending on personal preferences. The four primary
paths are *hatha* yoga, *jnana* yoga, *karma* yoga and *bhakti* yoga (see right).
Of these, the most recognized form practised in the West is *hatha* yoga
– from a Sanskrit word meaning the union of the sun (*ha*, representing
masculine energy) and the moon (*tha*, feminine energy) – which is an
umbrella term for many of the styles of yoga that we see on yoga-centre
schedules, such as Astanga and Sivananda yoga (see pp21–22). Although
most of the practices in this book are drawn from the *hatha* yoga path,
which teaches us how to balance our energy using asanas, pranayama,
concentration, meditation and cleansing practices, the pearls have been
written to embrace as many yogic paths as possible, for maximum appeal.
For example, as well as drawing on the four paths opposite, teachings
are included from *tantra* yoga, which places emphasis on tools such as
mantras, mudras, visualization and meditation to purify the mind as well as
the physical outer shell. We could, in fact, say that all yoga is *tantric* (the
Sanskrit word *tantra* meaning "to weave"), as it allows us to perceive how
closely spirit and matter – the warp and weft of life – are interwoven.

THE FOUR MAIN YOGA PATHS EXPLAINED

• **Hatha yoga** This path forms part of *raja* yoga, the "royal" path or path of kings, which employs meditation practices as a way of freeing the mind and attaining liberation. *Hatha* yoga follows the eight-limbed system recommended by the sage Patanjali in his *Yoga Sutras*, which includes, alongside psycho-physical exercises, cleansing practices and meditation (see pp14–15). *Hatha* yoga's main instrument is the body, which may be why this form of yoga has such great appeal to people in the West who are in search of enhanced health and well-being

• **Jnana yoga** The aim of this yogic path is to achieve a connection with the transcendent self through the study of yoga philosophy. The Sanskrit word *jnana* means "knowledge", especially spiritual knowledge, and the main tools of this path are self-study and enquiry. Jnana yoga tends to have particular appeal to people drawn to intellectual pursuits.

• **Karma yoga** The aim of this yogic path is to find a connection with the divine through selfless service to others – the Sanskrit word *karma* means "action", or work. Mother Teresa and Mahatma Gandhi are embodiments of this path of yoga, which often appeals to people who are drawn to charitable pursuits.

• **Bhakti yoga** This yogic path involves connecting with a mystical "otherness" through worship, ritual and song, all of which can touch the heart. The Sanskrit word *bhakti* means "devotion", or worship. This approach often appeals to people drawn to ritual and ceremony.

THE EIGHT-LIMBED PATH

The *Yoga Sutras* – one of the most influential hatha yoga texts of all time (see also p11) – was written by a Brahmin sage called Patanjali. Its 185 compressed axioms, or "threads of thought" in accordance with the meaning of the Sanskrit word *sutra*, set out practical ways to achieve

1 YAMA The first limb recommends five ethical practices or restraints (see below). This book offers ways to apply these "rules" to everything from your diet to your relations with other people.
• **Ahimsa**: applying non-violence to every part of your life; not harming others or yourself • **Satya**: truth, or living according to your own truth • **Asteya**: non-stealing • **Brahmacharya**: abstinence; containing sexual energy
• **Aparigraha**: non-grasping, or non-covetousness; letting go of desires.

2 NIYAMA The second limb prescribes five essential self-observances (see above right). This book offers guidance on how to put them into action through all sorts of exercises and meditations.
• **Saucha**: "cleanliness", both internal and external • **Santosha**: "contentment", or an acceptance of what life brings you
• **Tapas**: "austerity", or disciplined practice • **Swadhaya**: "self-study", the study of spiritual texts to promote understanding • **Ishwara pranidhana**: "surrender to a higher being".

3 ASANA The third limb refers to the physical yoga poses practised to prepare the body to sit in meditation – the Sanskrit word *asana* means "seat". Many poses are recommended in this book – practise them either one by one or as a sequence.

union with the divine by following a path that has eight progressive "limbs", or observances. The various elements of this eight-limbed path (see below) come up in different contexts throughout this book to help you to adopt a yogic approach to life both on and off your yoga mat.

4 PRANAYAMA The fourth limb is the art of breathing well. *Prana* means "breath", "vitality" or "energy", and *ayama* "to stretch". *Pranayama* regulates and extends energy flow through the body. You'll find a choice of exercises in this book, plus ways to apply them in poses.

5 PRATYAHARA The fifth limb means "to reverse" or draw in the mind and senses away from the outside world to induce calm. Techniques to achieve this are scattered throughout the book.

6 DHARANA The sixth limb urges you to concentrate, until your mind becomes focused on a still point. The Sanskrit root

dha means "to support", and the final two limbs (see below) rest on this one. There are concentration exercises in all chapters.

7 DHYANA *Dhyana* is the unbroken flow of consciousness toward one point of focus, or meditation. This limb is the fruit of *dharana*, occurring as you focus on one point in a state of continuous calm – the root *dhi* means "intellect" or "thinking".

8 SAMADHI Observing the first seven limbs brings you into a balanced mind-state, where you are aware of the eternal. *Sama* means "equal" and *dhi* "thinking".

THE YOGA BODY

Practising yoga not only enhances your physical body and fitness, but also purifies your energetic body. It does so by gradually unblocking your energy pathways, or *nadis*, so that your life-force, or *prana*, can flow freely with the aim of awakening your latent energy, known as *kundalini*. Many of the pearls in this book will encourage this process by cleansing the energy centres, known as chakras (see right), which lie along your main energy pathway, the *sushumna nadi*. Other pearls will guide you to cleanse the five *koshas*, or "envelopes of consciousness" (see p19). These are the body's subtle energy "sheaths" – five components like layers of an onion, which make up the human being: body, mind and spirit.

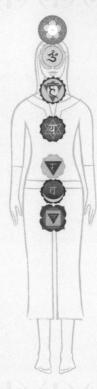

THE MAJOR CHAKRAS

Mooladhara chakra Located at the perineum, the floor of your torso, this, the root or base chakra, is the lowest chakra on the *sushumna nadi* that runs along your spine. The seat of primal energy, survival instincts and "base" drives, it is associated with the element earth and the colour red. *Kundalini*, or your latent store of psychic energy, is perceived to lie at this chakra, and is often depicted by an image of a coiled serpent (the coil represents the intensity of this energy). Many of the exercises in this book – including meditation and visualization techniques – begin to encourage this "sleeping serpent" to awaken, so that it can rise through and vitalize all of your chakras. To begin to experience the energy of your root chakra, turn to pearl 58 (see p56).

Swadhisthana chakra Located around your pubic bone or coccyx, this, the second chakra as you rise up the *sushumna*, is often referred to as the sacral chakra. Associated with the element water and the colour orange, it governs your sexuality and creativity. It is also thought to be the storehouse of your collective unconscious. To begin to experience the energy of your sacral chakra, turn to pearl 579 (see p232).

Manipura chakra Located behind your navel, this, the navel or solar plexus chakra, is your body's power centre. Associated with the element fire and the colour yellow, it governs your overall vitality, energy and drive. This chakra can also be thought of as your body's "business centre" because of its association with ego and worldly success. To begin to experience the energy of your navel chakra, turn to pearl 186 (see p98).

Anahata chakra Located in the centre of your chest, behind your heart, lies your heart chakra, often referred to as the "gateway to the void". Here your energy shifts from the "grosser" elements of the lower chakras to more subtle realms (its associated element is air, and its colours are pink and green). This is the seat of emotions and of "psychic sounds". To begin to experience the energy of your heart chakra, turn to pearl 450 (see p188).

Vishuddhi chakra Found behind the throat, the throat chakra is associated with self-expression and purification. Its associated element is ether, or space – the elements become increasingly refined as you move up the chakra system – and its colour is blue. To begin to experience the energy of the throat chakra, turn to pearl 728 (see p280).

Ajna chakra Your psychic command centre, this chakra is situated between the eyes, in the seat of the brain, and is often referred to as the third-eye chakra. Its colour is indigo. Your centre of intuition, governing sight on both the physical and spiritual planes, this chakra lies beyond the elements and the rules that govern the temporal world. To begin to experience the energy of the third-eye chakra, turn to pearl 973 (see p362).

Sahasrara chakra Emanating in all directions from the crown of the head is the highest of your energy centres, your crown chakra, which is associated with the colour violet. This is your threshold to the psychic and spiritual realms. To begin to experience the energy of the crown chakra, turn to pearl 997 (see p370).

Bindu This lesser-known energy point at the back of your head is sometimes referred to as the eighth chakra. To begin to sense your bindu, turn to pearl 999 (see p371).

THE FIVE KOSHAS

Yogic philosophy views the body as having five different energetic layers, known as sheaths or *koshas*, each expressing a different aspect of human existence. While only a few of the pearls in this book mention the koshas directly, many of them, from physical poses to meditation techniques, cleanse and vitalize these layers without you even being aware of it.

• **Annamaya kosha** This is the outer, physical layer or "sheath" of the body, or the "food body", which we see with our eyes and perceive with our conscious mind.

• **Pranamaya kosha** The next sheath, or layer of consciousness, is a more subtle one, which, although not visible to the eye, *is* perceived by the conscious mind. This layer regulates physiological processes, such as respiration, circulation and digestion.

• **Manamaya kosha** This is known as the lower mind, or lower intelligence, sheath. Operating on a subconscious level only, it is the layer of consciousness that thinks, feels, and stories memories and emotions.

• **Vijnanamaya kosha** Also operating on a subconscious level, this sheath, known as the higher intelligence body, represents the aspect of the mind that dreams, is aware of psychic experience and has increased clarity.

• **Anandamaya kosha** Known as the bliss sheath, this is the deepest, most spiritual aspect of your personality, where pure, meditative awareness exists.

MODERN STYLES OF HATHA YOGA

In ancient times, a seeker of yoga would sit, with dedication, on the doorstep of a yoga master until the teacher would agree to train him. Still today, there is a saying that the right teacher arrives when the student is ready. However, the numerous variations of hatha-yoga styles that have developed in the West in the last fifty years, each with a distinct emphasis and its own mix of mind and body techniques according to different teachers' approaches, can make it difficult to choose which "style" of yoga you want to follow in the first place.

Since yoga is about overall lifestyle, it's important to choose an approach that fits not only with your daily needs but also with your general preferences. To start your search for a style that suits you, it can be helpful to learn a little about the different styles of yoga that you might see detailed on a gym or yoga-centre schedule. The key styles are therefore outlined on pp21–22 – to give you a certain level of starter information on each one. The 1001 pearls of wisdom in the pages that follow present many inspiring methods from a wide range of these systems so that you can benefit from yoga in its broadest sense. As T.K.V. Desikachar said, *"Yoga ... comes from a vast and ancient source. The only authentic yoga is one which works for each person according to circumstances and needs, and there are many possibilities."*

STYLES OF HATHA YOGA EXPLAINED

Astanga Vinyasa yoga This was developed by Sri K. Pattabhi Jois (born 1915), a student of Sri Tirumalai Krishnamacharya (1888–1989). He set up a yoga school in the palace of his student, the Maharaja of Mysore, in 1924. Here, Pattabhi Jois teaches asanas as a gateway to the other seven limbs of yoga, as set out by the sage Patanjali (see pp14–15). This style of yoga involves practising dynamic postures in set flowing sequences, or *vinyasas*, to the rhythm of the breath. Postures are held for a count of up to 10 breaths, but often for fewer. Many contemporary styles of yoga have been modified from this pure system, including vinyasa flow and dynamic yoga.

Iyengar yoga Named after another teacher who studied under Krishnamacharya – B.K.S. Iyengar (born 1918), who is based in Pune, India – Iyengar yoga is a structural, posture-based approach to hatha yoga which concentrates on body alignment and is often used therapeutically to help those with health problems or disabilities. Precision work in physical postures is the meditative focus of the Iyengar system, which utilizes props, including blocks, chairs and belts. Poses are held for longer than in Pattabhi Jois's Astanga style.

Viniyoga Renowned yoga sage Krishnamacharya passed on the therapeutic yogic approach known as viniyoga – to his son, T.K.V. Desikachar (born 1938). In this style of yoga, teachers tailor programmes for the individual, carefully choreographing *vinyasas*, or sequences of postures, linked with breathing, that will enhance the well-being of that particular person. This yoga practice utilizes meditation, reflection, chanting and study as well as the posture work and relaxation common to all styles of hatha yoga.

Sivananda yoga One of the largest schools of yoga, this style was spread worldwide by Swami Vishnu-Devananda (1927–93), who studied under Swami Sivananda (1887–1963). Chanting, pranayama, poses and meditation form the basis of the practice, alongside the five pillars of yogic balance (see right), creating a yoga that relates to the whole person.

Satyananda yoga This style was founded by Swami Satyananda Saraswati (born 1923), who tailored the ancient energetic science of tantra yoga to meet the needs of modern life. He founded the first yoga university, the Bihar School of Yoga, in 1964, in Mungar, India.

Kundalini yoga This follows the tradition of Yogi Bhajan (born 1929), who came to the West from India in 1969. It focuses on raising *kundalini* (latent energy) to awaken the chakra energy centres (see pp16–18) with mantras, breathing exercises and meditation.

OTHER STYLES OF YOGA

Shadow yoga Developed by Shandor Remete, this form of hatha yoga works with the body's *marmas*, or vital pressure points that lie along the *nadi* energy channels.

Pure yoga and Anusara yoga Rod Stryker and John Friend respectively developed these styles, which employ varying degrees of the six "styles" on pp21–22.

Kripalu yoga This form of hatha yoga, developed by Swami Kripalu, celebrates the wisdom of the body and emphasizes proper breathing, alignment and concentration.

Scaravelli yoga Vanda Scaravelli, who studied with B.K.S. Iyengar, gave her name to this graceful approach, which embraces "waves" of energy to release tension.

THE FIVE PILLARS OF YOGIC BALANCE

The Sivananda school of yoga (see left) devised a model of five pillars that encourages us to acknowledge, understand and embrace all the elements essential for a balanced, healthy lifestyle – more detailed guidance on which is scattered throughout this book. Applying these five precepts in your life will help you to stay healthy, balanced and happy.

• **Right Exercise** This means regularly practising asanas, and other forms of exercise, with good intention and according to your age, state of health and the needs of your body.

• **Right Breathing** This involves working toward awareness of the breath at all times and re-establishing the deep, natural breathing of a child, which energizes your whole being (see pp34–35).

• **Right Thinking** This entails decluttering your mind of its many scattered thoughts to increase your sense of clarity and calm, and cultivating a positive attitude.

• **Right Nutrition** This means being aware of what you "feed" and fuel your body with – preferably a healthy range of fresh, seasonal, nutritious food in moderation – and eating that food slowly and mindfully at the appropriate times.

• **Right Relaxation** This entails taking time out to balance all the activity in your life with adequate rest to maintain a sense not only of physical relaxation but also mental, emotional and energetic relaxation, restoring and revitalizing your entire being.

WARM-UP SEQUENCES

In order to gain maximum benefit from any of the asanas featured in this book (each of which is marked by a symbol like this ➤), it's important to limber up before you begin. Limbering makes injury less likely by relieving stiffness, warming and lengthening your muscles, and increasing the circulation of your body fluids. It also makes you more aware of any energy blockages so that the asanas you do are more likely to clear your energy channels and enable prana to flow freely through your energy body. Perform these limbering exercises in sequence to bring the body's major joints and spine into alignment before asanas.

ANKLE AND WRIST ROTATIONS

1 Sit comfortably, so you can reach your feet – press each of your fingers between your toes, trying to separate and stretch them. Then rotate your ankle 5 times in each direction. Repeat on the other foot.

2 Now make your hands into fists and rotate your wrists 5 times in each direction. Finish by playing an imaginary piano with your fingers in the air.

HEAD AND SHOULDER ROLLS

1 Sit or stand comfortably and lower your chin down toward your chest. Carefully roll your head to one side – your ear toward your shoulder, and then roll to the other side, feeling your neck muscles ease out. Don't drop your head back. Repeat 5 times.

2 Inhaling, lift your shoulders toward your ears. Exhaling, roll them back and down. Repeat 5 times.

YOGA MUDRA SEQUENCE

1 Sit on the floor with your legs crossed, clasp your hands behind your back, interlink your fingers and stretch your arms back. Inhaling, look up. Exhaling, fold into a forward bend, taking your brow toward the ground. Take 5 full breaths. Then, inhaling, return to your starting position.

2 Place your hands on the floor behind you, fingers pointing forward. Lift your chest, arch your spine and carefully drop your head back (if your neck doesn't complain). Take 5 full breaths. Inhaling, return to your starting position.

3 Place your left hand on your right knee and your right hand on the floor behind you, then twist to the right and look over your right shoulder. Hold the position while you take 5 full breaths. Then return to the centre.

4 Place your right hand on your left knee and left hand on the floor behind you, then twist to the left. Hold the position for 5 full breaths. Then return to the centre.

To finish, open your mouth, reach your tongue toward your chin, exhale and look up with your eyes. This is Lion Pose (see pearl **27**).

HIP LIMBERS

1 Lie on your back and hug your right thigh into your belly. Exhaling, squeeze it. Inhaling, release your grasp and change legs. Do 5 repetitions on each leg. This is called *vatnyasana*, or Wind-relieving Pose (see pearl **782**).

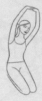

2 Kneel with your knees together and your buttocks resting on your heels. Reach your arms up, interlink your fingers and stretch up, holding for 5 breaths. Gently extend the stretch to the right, then the left.

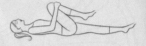

3 Still kneeling, place your hands on the floor behind you, fingers pointing forward. Press your chest up to create a gentle back-bend without compressing your lower back. Hold for 5 breaths if you can.

4 Roll your upper body forward, bringing your chest to your thighs and your forehead to the floor. Relax your arms by your sides. This is Child's Pose (see pearl **864**).

PREPARING FOR YOGA

In order to get the full benefits of a physical yoga practice – chiefly increased strength and flexibility of both body and mind, as well as an increased sense of focus and clarity – there are certain guidelines that you are recommended to follow.

- Aim for a 20-minute daily practice.
- Try to establish a fixed time for your practice every day. The ideal times are first thing in the morning (before you eat breakfast) and at twilight.
- Avoid eating for two hours before you practise.
- Find a clean, quiet, warm and well-ventilated place for your practice, with enough space to stretch your arms to the side and overhead.
- If you practise outside, choose a quiet, clean place away from the public gaze and direct sunlight.
- Wear loose comfortable clothing which stretches with your body and does not inhibit any movement. Natural fibres are best.
- Practise with bare feet, but keep some socks at hand to keep your feet warm in the final relaxation pose.
- Buy a yoga mat (from a yoga centre, sports shop or online) and invest in some yoga blocks and a yoga belt if you find them useful.
- Don't practise during the first two days of menstruation: Just relax and meditate. Thereafter, during menstruation, do gentle seated forward bending, hip-opening and restorative poses, such as Child's Pose, and keep your abdomen lower than your heart.
- If you are very stressed or depressed, it's best to avoid a rigorous yoga practice. Instead, opt for a range of gentle poses, breathing exercises and relaxation techniques.

SUN SALUTATION SEQUENCE

Traditionally, the Sun Salutation sequence of poses, or *Surya Namaskara*, was a prayer used to salute the sunrise. The sequence stretches your major muscles and cultivates concentration, giving you a sense of meditation in movement. Use it, after limbering, as a preparation for practising the poses in this book or as a sequence on its own at times of day when you

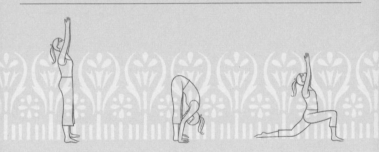

1 Stand with your feet firm and parallel, and your spine straight, arms by your side, in Mountain Pose. Breathe steadily. Inhaling, raise your arms overhead and look up.

2 Exhaling, dive slowly into a forward bend, planting your hands on either side of your feet. If your back is stiff, modify the pose by bending your knees.

3 Inhaling, look forward. Exhaling, lunge your left leg back, knee to the floor. Keep the right knee in a right angle. Inhaling, raise your arms and look up.

need to raise energy and stamina. The traditional sequence is composed of 12 postures woven on the breath, but there are many versions of the practice. The version given here, while softer than some, includes two lunges (steps 3 and 8), which increases it from 12 to 14 steps. These lunges help to ease the transition from forward bend to plank pose.

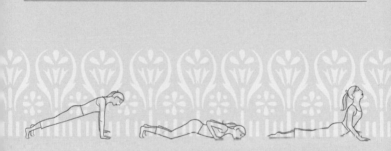

4 Exhaling, place your hands beside your front foot and step the foot back to create a plank shape with your body. Keep your feet hip-width apart.

5 Without taking a breath, lower your chin, chest and knees to the floor, with your chest between your hands – as a transition to the next posture.

6 Inhaling, straighten your legs, top of the toes facing down, and press on your hands to arch your spine into Upward Dog. Try to keep your neck long.

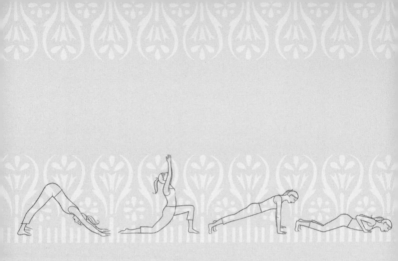

7 Exhaling, press on your hands, straighten your arms and push your hips backward and upward, into Downward Dog. Try to push your heels to the ground. Take 5 breaths in and out.

8 Inhaling, lunge your left foot forward, this time lowering your right knee to the floor. Keep your front knee in a right angle. Raise your arms toward the sky and look up.

9 Exhaling, step your left foot back to create a plank shape again (as in step 4).

10 Without taking a breath, lower chin, chest and knees to the floor, as in step 5.

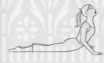

11 Inhaling, straighten your legs and push on your hands to arch your spine.

12 Exhaling, push your hips back and toward the sky. Take 5 breaths in and out.

13 Inhaling, step your feet between your hands, keeping your feet hip-width apart. Exhaling, fold your head toward your shins and release your spine, bending your knees if necessary.

14 Inhaling, come back to initial standing pose, feet hip-width apart, and reach your arms in a wide circle to end with them above your head. Exhaling, return them to your sides.

PREPARING TO MEDITATE

Meditation, or *dhyana*, the seventh of hatha yoga's eight stages (see pp14–15), is an important part of yoga – particularly in your quest for right thinking and right relaxation (see p23). Regular meditation practice brings about a state of mind fully in the present, which allows you to observe your thought processes without being distracted by a scattered mind. Don't feel put off when your mind is darting from thought to thought or emotion to emotion. If you keep watching yourself and gently clearing your mind, it will eventually become like a vast, calm ocean. The art is to learn to dip into this oceanic awareness more and more as time goes on – to reach a pure awareness of simply being. Many of the yoga "pearls" in this book explore ways of cultivating this meditative state but it's important to know the basics, such as practice tips and the key postures, before exploring any of the techniques explained:

Meditation tips

- Set a fixed time for practice each day: best is upon rising in the morning or before bed.
- Practise before eating, so you are not distracted by the digestive process.
- Begin with 10–15 minutes' practice every day, and build up the time slowly.
- Designate a clean, quiet, well-ventilated room for your practice.
- Wear warm, loose clothing and place a blanket or rug underneath you.
- If you tend to fall asleep, have a refreshing shower before you practise.

MEDITATIVE SITTING POSTURES

Easy Pose *Sukhasana*

This is the traditional meditation pose. *Sukha* means "ease", but if you feel any discomfort, sit on a yoga block or folded blanket.

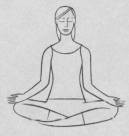

1 Sit cross-legged on the bony part of your buttocks and lift your spine as straight as possible. Place your hands on your knees, palms facing upward.
2 Close your eyes and relax your entire body, while maintaining alertness in your spine.

Thunderbolt Pose *Vajrasana*

Vajra means "thunderbolt" and refers to the energy channel, *vajra nadi*, that links the genito-urinary nerve pathway to the brain, inducing spiritual awareness. This pose suits meditation because it keeps the spine and *vajra nadi* alert and awake.

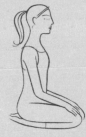

1 Kneel with knees together, a yoga block or folded blanket beneath your sitting bones if desired. Anchor your sitting bones well.
2 Stretch the front of your ankles and toes, and point your heels up. Rest your palms on your thighs. Close your eyes and maintain alertness.

THE IMPORTANCE OF THE BREATH

"Good" breathing is of paramount importance not only for a balanced yoga practice (see box below) but also for a healthy, balanced life in general (see p23). All too often, we breath in a quick, shallow way (into our chest only rather than our belly), making full use neither of all our breathing muscles nor of our lung capacity. Such sustained "bad" breathing can eventually lead to physical tension and a whole range of other problems, so it's important to become aware of the breath and return to our natural, deep way of breathing (like that of a child), which is supremely healing and balancing. The exercise opposite is the perfect way to start doing this; it's best to get used to the feeling of *this* technique before doing any of the exercises suggested in this book.

BREATHING IN POSTURES

When practising the yoga asanas suggested in this book, aim to breath in and out through your nose, keeping the rhythm even and unforced. If it helps you to focus on your breath, imagine it as blue ink spreading throughout your body and into each cell – being sure that the "Ink" (your fresh in-take of oxygen) reaches as many parts of your body as possible to nourish them with fresh energy. Remain mindful of your breathing the whole time.

THREE-PART YOGA BREATHING

This exercise encourages full, deep breathing. Once you have mastered it lying down with your hands to guide you, aim to apply it to your everyday breathing so that long, full, easy breathing becomes second nature. Then also explore it as you practise yoga asanas.

1 Lie down with your knees bent up and your feet hip-width apart on the floor. Place a firm folded blanket beneath your head if it feels comfortable, to encourage neck length.

2 Rest your hands just below your navel. Observe your breathing for 10 full breaths, drawing each one deep into your belly. Feel your navel rise each time you inhale and fall each time you exhale.

3 Now rest your hands on your rib-cage and observe your breathing again for 10 breaths. As your lungs empty at the end of each exhalation, feel your middle fingers touch. As your lungs fill on each inhalation, feel your fingers separate. At the end of the tenth breath, aim to empty your lungs completely and feel your navel draw toward your spine.

4 Now rest your hands across your collar-bones, letting your elbows rest to the sides. As you inhale, feel your chest rise and your collar-bones expand toward the sides of the room. Become aware of fresh space between your shoulder-blades. As you exhale, relax your chest, empty your lungs and feel your navel draw toward your spine.

5 Finally, practise steps 1–3 so that you breathe into all three portions of your torso: your belly, your rib-cage and your collar-bones. This is three-part yoga breathing. Try to keep each inhalation and exhalation of equal length. Follow the flow of the breath, imagining each one as a wave washing through you. Then feel how your steady, calm breathing makes your mind, too, feel like a still but powerful sea.

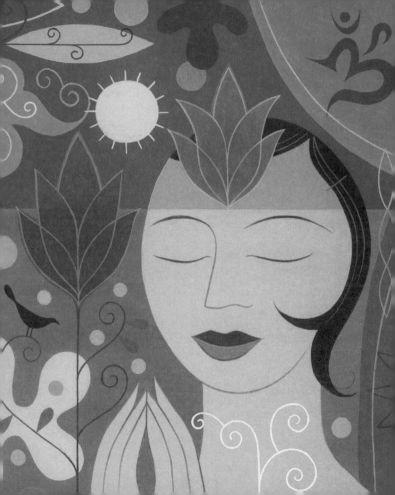

STARTING YOUR DAY WELL

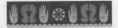

AWAKENING NATURALLY

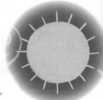

1   **MORNING REMEMBRANCE** *"Yoga: an ancient practice, a complete way of life."*
INDIAN PROVERB

2   **Shelter your senses** Closing down the senses, a practice called *pratyahara*, brings about great peace. Wearing an eye mask in bed shuts out external distractions during sleep, allowing you to wake to each day more fully refreshed.

3   **Greet the day gently** Give up your harsh-trilled alarm clock and invest in one that wakes you to a humming bird or dawn chorus. Yoga encourages you to remember daily that you're part of nature. Even better, try to awaken naturally. Before bed, practise **Exhalation breathing (982)**. As you finish, repeat out loud the time at which you would like to wake the next morning.

4   **STAYING AWAKE NATURALLY** *"We must learn to reawaken and keep ourselves awake, not by mechanical aid but by an infinite expectation of the dawn."*
HENRY DAVID THOREAU (1817–1862), USA

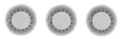

5   **Deep breathing** Yoga philosophy teaches that we are allocated
only a certain number of breaths between our first inhalation at
birth and our last exhalation at death. So the more slowly you
draw each breath, the longer – and calmer – you will live.

---

6   **RESPECT EACH BREATH**
"If you breathe well, you will live long on the earth."
INDIAN PROVERB

---

7   **Unspoken prayer** The natural sound of your breath is like a
prayer welcoming you to the day. On waking, become aware
of your breathing before you do anything else. Notice how the
inhalation makes the sound *SO*. Then, as you exhale, notice how
it makes the sound *HAM* (or *"hum"*). In Sanskrit, *soham* means
"He am I" – "He" refers to God, or the
creative force of nature, so your breath links
you with the divine. For centuries, yogic
sages have explained that this unconscious
repetitive prayer (*ajapa japa*) goes on
continuously within every living creature.

[039]

8   **The creation mantra** Before you get out of bed, cradle yourself in the sound that yogis believe brought the universe into being by chanting *OM* (pronounced "aum"). Take a deep breath in. As you exhale with an open mouth, let the sound "aaa" well up from deep in your belly, round your lips to make the sound "uuu", then close your lips to finish with a soft "mmm". Repeat until you feel awake and really alive.

9   **Think about the One** Before you get up, contemplate this saying from Vedic times (see p10): *"I and the source are one."* The journey of yoga involves remembering that everything in the universe emanates from a single energy source. Yoga asanas, pranayama and meditation bring you an awareness of this unity.

10   **Guided thinking** To gain further insight into the yogic notion of unity, think about this phrase from the ancient text *Yogavasistha Maharamayana: "The same undivided and indivisible space is outside and inside of a thousand pots. Likewise the Self pervades all beings."*

11   **Simply stretch** Yoga teaches that since the earth moves constantly, so too should your body's energy – even when lying in bed in the morning. As soon as you wake, stretch your limbs like a starfish to get the energy flowing for the day ahead.

12   **Tapping the heavenly drum** Your senses tend to withdraw into your body at nighttime. To "retune" your hearing in the morning, sit up and close your eyes, press your index fingers into your ears, closing the flaps, and lightly tap your index fingernails with the tips of your third fingers for 1 minute. Enjoy the inner drumming.

13   **Think positive** A *sankalpa* is a phrase in the present tense to fix your mind on positive action. Say to yourself in the morning, "I am vibrant! I am ready for anything that the day brings."

14   **Positive visualization** Decide on an affirmation, such as, "I am truly awake." Close your eyes and imagine writing these words slowly in vibrant red ink. Let them soak in. Then write them again quickly many times in bright yellow ink before opening your eyes. This mantra will help your intention to become a reality.

15   **A natural step** Yoga offers a ladder by which you can climb out of everyday boundaries into *jivanmukti*, liberation in life. Stepping out of bed with positive intention is the first rung on the ladder.

16   **STEPPING INTO AWARENESS** *"The distance is nothing; it is only the first step that is difficult."*
MADAME MARIE DU DEFFAND (1697–1780), FRANCE

17   **Fully alert** The word *buddha* translates as someone who is fully awake, or enlightened. A *buddha* experiences the eighth limb of yoga, known as *samadhi* (see p15), meaning self-realization or union with the divine. As you begin your day, remember that this state of mind is accessible to anyone who desires it with sincerity. Start by simply trying to be aware in every moment.

18   **Are you awake?** The teaching tool of one *swami* (Indian religious teacher) was to repeat the phrase "Are you awake?" at certain points throughout the day. This reminded his students to remain mindful and not to slip into sleepy patterns of habit. Repeat it to yourself every now and again.

19   **CLEAN BODY, PURE MIND**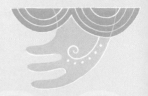

"Krishna insisted on outer cleanliness and inner cleansing. Clean clothes and clean minds are an ideal combination."

SRI SATHYA SAI BABA (BORN 1926), INDIA

20   **Refreshing tonic** After showering or bathing, splash your face, hands and feet with revitalizing cold water to stimulate the many nerve endings, reawakening your sense of touch.

21   **PURIFYING PLUNGE**

"Wash away, Waters, whatever sin is in me, what wrong I have done, what imprecation I have uttered, and what untruth I have spoken."

RIG VEDA (c.1500–600BCE), INDIA

22   **Revitalizing splash** A swim is a wonderful way to awaken your senses and stretch out your limbs in the morning. Let the rhythm of the swimming strokes calm your thoughts and any anxieties. Stilling your thought waves in this way is the essence of yoga.

23   **Wake up your mouth** Since your mouth is considered in yogic anatomy to be the gateway to your body, it is important to clean it early in the morning. Ayurveda, the ancient system of Indian healing, recommends traditional Indian cleansing products, which are often based on neem. Buy them from a health-food store; alternatively, rub your teeth with the rind of a lemon, which removes tarnishing, then use the juice to clean your teeth.

24   **FLAWLESS NATURE** *"Unto the pure all things are pure."*
THE EPISTLE OF PAUL TO TITUS 1.15

25   **Cleanse your tongue** *Jihva moola dhauti*, tongue-cleansing, is an important part of a yogi's morning routine. The coating on the tongue comprises impurities rejected by the body that can act as a breeding ground for bacteria. Take a teaspoon, stick out your tongue and gently scrape the surface. It only takes a minute.

26   **Nasal cleansing** Yogis around the world like to cleanse their sinuses the traditional Indian way once a month or at the onset of a cold. To follow suit, buy a neti pot online and fill it with lukewarm water containing a sprinkle of sea salt. Tilt your head to one side, insert the spout into one nostril and let the water pour through your sinus passages until it drips out of the other nostril. Repeat on the other side. Do not snort or force the process.

27 **Lion Pose** *Simhasana* Best performed in the morning, this cleansing practice is said to purify the tongue and prevent halitosis. Kneel with your buttocks on your heels and your back straight. Place your hands face down on your knees, spreading your fingers like lion's claws, and straighten your arms. 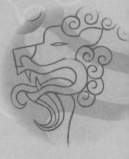 Stretch your mouth open as wide as you can, and, as you exhale, stick out your tongue, reaching it toward your chin. Look up with your eyes and hold the pose for as long as is comfortable. Inhale and repeat 3–5 times. Then relax. **>** 45

28 **ABSORB EARTH ENERGY** *"Take the breath of the new dawn and make it part of you. It will give you strength."*
HOPI SAYING

A SENSE OF OPENING

29   **Mudra for receptivity** *Pushpaputa Mudra* To create a feeling
of inner spaciousness and abundance that will last throughout
your day, make this symbolic gesture, the Sanskrit name of which
translates as "handful of flowers". Kneel with your buttocks on
your heels and place the backs of your hands on your thighs or
knees, fingers pointing diagonally toward each other. Let each
palm form an an open cup shape, resting your thumbs against
your index fingers. Close your eyes and visualize, with pristine
clarity, your hands filled with beautiful flowers and abundance.

30   **Cultivate awareness** Early in the morning, spend a minute scanning your body, checking how you feel today. Yoga teaches us that what we feel, and how we project it, creates our reality. Simply being aware of how you feel therefore alters the way you connect with the world around you. Decide to interact with people positively today and to open your mind to new experiences.

31   **NEW DAY DAWNS** *"Only that day dawns to which we are awake."*
HENRY DAVID THOREAU (1817–1862), USA

32   **Opening to ethics** The five *yamas* – moral ethics that ultimately cross all cultures and creeds – lie at the foundation of the eight limbs of yoga defined by Patanjali (see p14). As you prepare for your day, spend a few moments contemplating one of the most important of them – *ahimsa*, or non-violence. Are there any issues you need to address to meet the requirements of this *yama*?

---

33   **BE READY TO ACCEPT THE GIFT**
"Yoga is the giver of untold happiness."
BHAGAVAD GITA (400–300BCE), INDIA

34   **Ponder connections** The Sanskrit root of the word *yoga*, *yuj*,
means "to yoke" or connect, drawing attention to the fact that
we are not isolated individuals, but share a connection with
everything that is. Before you head out into the world this
morning, spend a few minutes allowing this fact to sink into
your mind by repeating the mantra, *Tat tvam asi*: "Thou art that."

---

35   **EXPAND YOUR MIND**
*"It is you that pervades this universe, and this
universe exists in you. Your true nature is pure
Consciousness. Don't be small-minded."*
ASHTAVAKRA GITA (800–400BCE), INDIA

---

36   **Out of the groove** Just as the indentations of a vinyl record
predict its playing, yoga teaches that the mind is imprinted with
samskaras, behaviour patterns conditioned by our culture, life
experience, education and belief system. Asanas, pranayama and
meditation encourage us to explore these habits and to replace
limiting patterns with healthier ones. Start this process today
by observing the way you think about and respond to events.

37 **Cultivate "the watcher"** As you move around your home in the morning, look out of the windows and contemplate the outside world. Recognize that you're a player in a drama that is being created right now. Choose your part wisely and embrace it, yet cultivate a sense of detachment to transcend limitations.

38 **SELECT YOUR ROLE** *"We are responsible for what we are, and whatever we wish ourselves to be, we have the power to make ourselves. If what we are now has been the result of our past actions, it certainly follows that whatever we wish to be in the future can be produced by our present actions; so we have to know how to act."* SWAMI VIVEKANANDA (1863–1902), INDIA

39 **Regularity breeds receptivity** As you plan your diary, aim to build in a period of yoga practice at the same time every day.

40 **YOGA FOR TODAY** *"Yoga is not an ancient myth buried in oblivion. It is the most valuable inheritance of the present. It is the essential need of today and the culture of tomorrow."* SWAMI SATYANANDA SARASWATI (BORN 1923), INDIA

41   **Leap to the second rung** In Patanjali's eight-runged ladder of yoga (see pp14–15), the second stage is *niyama*, "laws" of personal conduct. To tune into these healthy life attitudes, spend a minute each time you begin asana practice considering the *niyama* known as *tapas* – intensity of discipline through practice.

42   **RIGHT THINKING** *"In truth it matters less what we do in practice than how we do it and why we do it."*
DONNA FARHI (BORN 1959), NEW ZEALAND

43   **Between postures** Resting between asanas allows you to become more receptive in your yoga as it gives time for both your body and your mind to process the effects, whether physical, mental or emotional, of each movement. In your morning practice, rest in **Child's Pose (864)** after postures you find challenging, observing the flow of your breath, in and out.

44   **AFTER REST WE FLOURISH** *"Take rest; a field that has rested gives a bountiful crop."*
OVID (43BCE–c.17CE), ROME

CAT POSE

Bidalasana

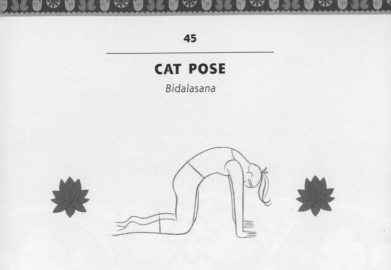

This pose stretches the core of the body, so is a good way to start your day. Think of its namesake, the cat (*bidala*), when gracefully arching your spine.

On all fours, place your hands beneath your shoulders, knees below your hips. Lengthen your spine. Inhaling, lift your tail-bone, dip your waist, stretch your throat and look up. Exhaling, round your spine and curl your tail-bone under (see above), drawing your chin in and your navel to your spine. Coordinate the movements with your breathing for 10 breaths. Then relax. > 46

46   **Cat Pose variation** To stretch the sides of your body, position yourself with a wall to your left and come into a table-top shape as if beginning **Cat Pose (45)**. Extend your right leg in a backward diagonal line from your hip. Root down into the ground with the outer edge of your right foot. Then twist to the right, bringing your back against the wall. Open your chest and, with your right shoulder stacked over your left, stretch your right arm above your head. Take 5–10 breaths, engaging the core muscles in your abdomen. Return to the table-top position for 2 breaths, repeat on the left side (with the wall on your right), then relax. **>** 57

47   **Awaken to your own truth** The second of the five *yamas*, yoga's moral ethics, is *satya*, or truth (see p14). See if you can intuit insights into your own nature as you do your yoga practice. In yoga, truth is not something that you learn, like knowledge, but is something that is revealed, like wisdom.

48   **OPEN UP AND WAIT** *"Be as a cup, and the universe flows into you. Be as an arrow, and the universe retreats from you."*
ZEN PROVERB

THE IMPORTANCE OF GROUNDING

49   **SEND DOWN ROOTS** *"For a tree to become tall it must grow tough roots among the rocks."*
FRIEDRICH NIETZSCHE (1844–1900), GERMANY

50   **Lotus visualization** Since ancient times, yogis have used the rich symbolism of the lotus flower to anchor meditation and to help to visualize physical postures. Stand tall and imagine yourself as a lotus, your pristine head rising high. Look down to see your firm, supportive stem (body and legs), held in place by strong roots (your feet), which draw nourishment from the earth.

51   **Connect to your roots** To start your day in a state of balanced groundedness, stand with your feet hip-width apart and explore how it feels to root downward into what yogis refer to as the "corners" of your feet – the joints of your big toes, the edges of your little toes, the backs of your heels (imagine you are wearing horseshoes), and the inner and outer sides of your heels.

52   **Foot massage** For stiff feet, slide your fingers between your toes and roll them like waves; then rotate each foot at the ankle joint.

53   **Foot energy** The feet are the site of a minor chakra that gathers in and distributes energy, which enables you to step out into the world and interact effectively with other people. To call in energy that often settles here during the night, explore your feet with Ankle Rotations (see step 1 of p24), **Foot massage (52)** and standing poses such as **Mountain Pose (57)**.

54   **Thirsty feet** When you do a morning asana practice, imagine that the arches of your feet are drawing up energy from the earth to quench their thirst. Urge your feet to direct this energy up your legs toward your pelvis to help to steady you throughout the day.

55   **Grounding energy lock** To activate what yogis might refer to as the "inner ankles", lift the inner arches of your feet when you're standing. This is *Pada Bandha*: an energy seal for the feet. Feel how it energizes not only your standing poses but also your gait: it will give you a spring in your step as you walk.

56   **STAND TALL TO RELAX** *"On every mountain height is rest."*
JOHANN WOLFGANG VON GOETHE (1749–1832), GERMANY

MOUNTAIN POSE

Tadasana

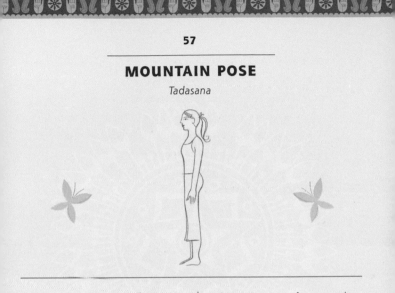

This pose evokes the stillness, strength and innate power of a mountain (*tada*), grounding the body and bringing a positive charge of energy.

Stand with your feet parallel and hip-width apart, grounding them through the base of your toes and heels. Keep your pelvis stable and neutral. Stretch through the sides of your body upward, keeping your shoulders down and arms relaxed by your sides. Lengthen the back of your neck and gaze at a point in front. Listen to your breathing for 5–10 deep breaths. Then relax. ➤ 98

58 **Feel your base chakra** The lowest energy centre on the chakra framework in humans (see p17) is *mooladhara*, the base chakra (*moola* means "root" and *adhara*, "substratum" or "base"). Close your eyes and take your focus to your pelvic floor, the site of this chakra. Breathe into the area for several minutes. This will tune you into its earthing energy and help you to express your needs.

59 **Base chakra mantra** The *bija mantra*, or seed sound, of the base chakra is *LAM* (pronounced "lum"). Sit upright with your spine straight and focus on your pelvic floor. Visualize the colour red, then gently sing the seed sound *LAM*. Gaze at its Sanskrit form in the centre of the chakra's visual representation (see above right). Feel the primal energy of this chakra and allow it to form a springboard for your day's action.

60   **Mooladhara yantra meditation** Sitting quietly, let your
eyes settle on the base chakra's *yantra*, or geometric form
(see below left). Breathing gently, let the vibrant energy of the
four large lotus petals empower you, and imagine the solid
square earthing you with its stability. Finally, let the red triangle
point you down toward the vast store of latent energy that lies
at the base of your spine, waiting to be awakened.

61   **Hand energy** Like your feet, your hands are the site of a minor
chakra that gathers in and distributes energy – in this case, the
energy that equips you to reach out to others. Activate it before
leaving home by stretching your digits, playing an imaginary piano
and circling your wrists first in one direction, then the other.

62   **Absorb earth energy** In a morning *asana* practice, imagine
that your hands are suction cups in poses such as **Cat Pose (45)**
and **Downward Dog Pose (481)**, drawing energy from the earth.

63   **EARTH WISDOM** *"... speak to the earth, and it shall teach thee."*
THE BOOK OF JOB 12.8

64   **Squatting** Stand with your feet hip-width apart, exhale and descend into a squat, dropping your pelvis between your heels as far as possible. This is a natural sitting position for many yogis and helps the feet to connect with the ground. Try it before using the lavatory in the morning – it can encourage elimination.

65   **SOLID GROUND** *"The foot feels the foot when it feels the ground."*
THE BUDDHA (c.563–c.483BCE), INDIA

66   **Partner squat** Doing a trust exercise with your partner in the morning sets you up well for encounters with other people later in the day. Stand facing each other at arm's distance, then grasp each other's wrists. Take a deep breath in. As you exhale, descend into a squat together, keeping your backs straight. To return to standing, inhale in unison, then push up through your feet.

67   **THE IMPORTANCE OF TRUST** *"Few things help an individual more than to place responsibility upon him, and to let him know that you trust him."*
BOOKER T. WASHINGTON (1856–1915), USA

68 **Sink into a pure heart** An Indian *swami* told the tale of a man who asked a yoga disciple, "Where can I find a place to discipline myself to understand my spirit?" The disciple replied, "That place lies in the pure and honest spirit where there is no false vanity." Try to connect with this sense of honesty and integrity within yourself each morning to infuse your day with a sense of purity.

69 **Alternate Nostril Breathing** *Anuloma Viloma* This calming technique stabilizes your energy levels at the start of the day by regulating the flow of energy through your body's main subtle energy channels (see p16). Sit with your spine straight, resting your hands on your thighs, palms facing upward. Take a few deep breaths to centre yourself. Inhale through both nostrils, then raise your left thumb to depress your left nostril. Exhale slowly through your right nostril. Relax your left hand and inhale through both nostrils. Raise your right thumb and close your right nostril. Exhale slowly through your left nostril, then relax your right hand and inhale through both nostrils. Repeat up to 12 breaths (6 on each side), aiming to lengthen each exhalation until it becomes twice the length of the inhalation.

70   **Supportive energy lock** *Bandha* is Sanskrit for "gate" or "lock". *Moola Bandha,* at the site of *mooladhara* chakra, around your pelvic floor (see p17), is the first of the three main energetic locks. Applying this helps to set your inner foundations at the start of the day, stabilizing your body and providing a sense of unshakeability on which to build your day's activities. To do this, lift your pelvic floor without contracting your abdominal muscles, and hold as you inhale. Exhale and release. Repeat several times.

71   **Energy visualization** The Sanskrit word *kundala* refers to the coil of a rope, and the term *kundalini* describes a coiled female serpent, a symbol of divine energy. Sitting comfortably, close your eyes and visualize her lying coiled at the base of your spine, near *mooladhara* chakra, the grounding energy centre. The aim of yoga practice is eventually (with a teacher's guidance) to rouse this symbolic sleeping serpent so she rises up the spine, vitalizing the chakras.

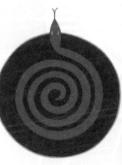

72   **Taking root to fly** As well as grounding yourself at the start of the day, it's important to embody grounding's opposing force, ascension. To do this, stand with your feet hip-width apart and try to gain a sense of drawing up your thigh muscles and knee caps, while your pelvis (your centre of gravity) stays firmly on top of your legs, like Stonehenge. Relax your spine and lift your rib-cage up and out of your pelvis. Feel how the experience of grounding and ascending simultaneously brings a sense of renewed energy.

73   **DUAL FOCUS** *"Heaven is under our feet as well as over our heads."*
HENRY DAVID THOREAU (1817–1862), USA

74   **Attach skyhooks** Each time you step outside today, imagine a hook at your breast-bone lifts your heart within your rib-cage, and another at the crown of your head connects you to the sky.

75   **Drop anchor** As you stroll down the street, picture your tail-bone as a great kangaroo's tail or your body as a ship drawing an anchor into port. This brings your pelvis into a safe, "neutral" position, neither tilted too far forward nor arched too far back.

ENCOURAGING VITALITY

76   **Early start** Yogis tend to get active even before taking breakfast, in order to kickstart their day with a sense of natural energy. The traditional way is with the Sun Salutation (*Suryanamaskara*): a series of linked yoga postures coordinated with your breathing that form a whole-body prayer to the sun (see pp28–31).

Exercise in the shower (77) Stretch your arms overhead in a full-body extension if you can't find the time for Sun Salutation on a really busy morning. It's better than nothing!

78   **Vital essence** *Sattwa* is the term for a state, or *guna*, of balance, as opposed to one of *rajas* (over-activity) or *tamas* (inertia). Aim to nourish yourself in a *sattwic* way each day by eating fresh, seasonal fruit and nourishing seeds.

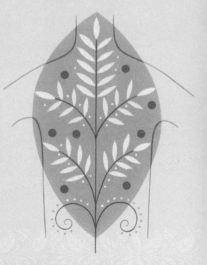

79   YOGIC ENERGY FOODS
"Foods that are tasty, wholesome and satisfying, that give long life, vitality, strength, health, happiness and satisfaction."
BHAGAVAD GITA (400–300BCE), INDIA

---

80   Foods of the yogis To maintain maximum energy, balance the food on your plate into ¼ protein (such as eggs or beans), ¼ carbohydrate (such as quinoa) and ½ fresh vegetables.

81   Bright breakfast Enjoy at least three vibrant-hued foods at breakfast, such as sliced melon, berries and kiwi in your cereal.

82   Wake-up drink Many modern yogis begin the day with reviving "yogi" tea (available from health-food stores), a nutrient-packed smoothie or the juice of half a lemon in a mug of hot water.

83   Caffeine fix? Try to avoid artificial stimulants, such as coffee, instead stimulating the body with asanas and pranayama. If you can't do without, try to really enjoy just one cup a day.

84   **Boost digestive energy** *Samana prana* is the "vital air", or energetic force, in the abdomen, which balances digestion (*sama* means "equal", "even" or "upright") and which carries vital nutrients throughout the body. Stress can disrupt its functioning, so make sure your breakfast time is calm, rather than snacking on the run.

85   **Eating meditation** Eat slowly and mindfully, enjoying each mouthful with all your senses rather than gulping it down. Yogis recommend chewing each bite 20–30 times before swallowing to allow your body to take advantage of the vital energy in food.

86   **Ethical awareness** Set up a yogic frame of mind for the day by tuning into three of the S's that form the yoga *yama* (ethics) and *niyama* (self-observances; see p14): *saucha*, **Inner cleanliness (87)**; *santosha*, **Contentment (88)**; and *satya*, **Seeking truth (89)**.

87   **Inner cleanliness** *Saucha* means cleanliness of mind as well as of body. Start the day using a soap with a scent that awakens your senses – try vibrant citrus, ginger or peppermint.

88   **Contentment** *Santosha* is the peaceful happiness that develops
as you learn to accept and love yourself. To start the day a more
vital person, give thanks for what you have and who you are.

89   **Seeking truth** *Satya* is knowing your own truth. Spend a few
moments in contemplation in the morning, connecting with your
innate sense of yourself. This will help to fire your encounters
with others throughout the day with an authentic energy.

90   **Self-truth mantra** The throat chakra's *bija mantra*, or seed
sound, *HAM* (pronounced "hum") fills the mind with vibrations
that remove obstacles currently limiting your self-expression. Sing
it quietly if thoughts hold you back in the morning, if you fear
criticism or if you tend to over-analyze the results of your actions.

---

91   **THE ENERGY OF TRUE YOGA**
*"Your mind will be secure in self-knowledge and
undisturbed by the voices of doctrine and ritual.
Then you will have achieved true yoga."*
BHAGAVAD GITA (400–300BCE), INDIA

92   **Tapping into divine energy** The abundant natural energy deep within us all is thought in yoga to be divine in essence – whether you think of it as emanating from a supreme being or from nature. All forms of yoga allow you to experience this energy.

93   **Touch your vital centre** The spiritual leader Osho (1931–1990) taught that everyone has the potential during yoga to "touch" the centre of existence. This ignites vitality in every part of you.

---

94   **INNER ENERGY**
"Yoga is not attained through the lotus posture and not by gazing at the tip of the nose. Yoga ... is the identity of the psyche with the transcendental Self."
KULA ARNAVA TANTRA (1000–1400CE), INDIA

---

95   **Opposite energies** When dressing, consider the yogic belief that the left side of your body signifies your intuitive, feminine energy and your right side your logical, masculine qualities. The Hindu god Prajapati embodied both polarities. Can you recognize both masculine and feminine qualities within yourself?

96   **Self-knowledge mudra** *Jnana Mudra* To start the day feeling engaged with the tasks ahead, sit with your spine straight and your hands on your knees, palms upward. Outstretch your fingers, like starfish. Now curl the index fingers in to touch the tips of your thumbs. Your index finger signifies your ego – the self that separates you from the universe – and your thumb the cosmic Self. Imagine the small self melting into the greater Self, absorbing its wise energy.

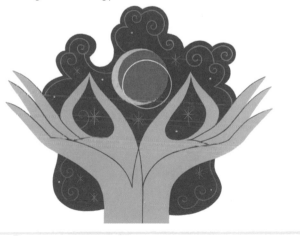

97   **Play your instrument** Yehudi Menuhin said of yoga, "Reduced to our own body, our first instrument, we learn to play it, drawing from it maximum resonance and harmony." When you do asanas, think of your body as a harp and each movement as a note being played. Let energy flow through your tuned strings.

98   **Chair Pose** *Utkatasana* This posture strengthens and enlivens the lower body so is useful in the morning if you have to spend much of the day sitting at a desk. Place your feet hip-width apart and parallel, gripping a yoga block or thick book between your thighs to enliven the inner "seams" of your legs. Bend your knees as if skiing, with your knees directly over your toes (block still in place). Swing your arms skyward and take 5–10 deep breaths, focusing your gaze on a fixed point in front of you. Then relax. ▶ 117

99   **Chair Pose vinyasa** For a quick boost before you begin working at a desk, crouch in **Chair Pose (98)**, without the yoga block, and practise the following flowing movements. Exhaling, reach your arms forward until you fold into a forward bend. Inhaling, sweep your arms up and sit back to Chair Pose. Repeat 5 times.

100   **Golden visualization** Lie on your back, breathe deeply and focus on your spine. Bring your attention to the left side of your body and try to tune into how it's feeling. Then do the same on the right side. Does one side feel more depleted of energy than the other? If so, visualize that side being bathed in glowing, golden energy for a few moments, then open your eyes.

101   **Energy of the day** Yoga teaches that there are three *gunas*, or energy forces, that inhabit all matter. *Rajas* is the active energy of the early part of day, of spring and of youth. This makes up a cycle with *sattwa*, balance, and *tamas*, inertia. Think how you can benefit from the active force *rajas* today – to pitch a new idea, for example, or simply to adopt a can-do attitude.

   Start the day shining (102) Cultivate *tejas*, Sanskrit for "lustre" or "majesty", with **Victorious Breath (527)**.

---

103   **REVEAL YOUR INNER VIBRANCY**
   "By cutting away sorrow,
   the brilliant light of the Self dawns."
   PATANJALI'S *YOGA SUTRAS* (300–200BCE), INDIA

EMBRACING FLUIDITY

104   THE POWER OF WATER *"Nothing in the world is more flexible and yielding than water. Yet when it attacks the firm and the strong, none can withstand it, because they have no way to change it. So the flexible overcome the adamant, the yielding overcome the forceful."*
LAO TZU (c.604–c.531BCE), CHINA

105   Your sacral chakra Explore the flowing energy of the sacral chakra (see p17) and of water, its associated element, when you get a chance to sit or lie in mid-morning relaxation. Simply close your eyes and vizualize a stream flowing into a deep lake in your pelvis. Feel the fluidity of this energy giving you the flexibility to respond creatively to situations and to see potential in others.

106   Mantra for flow *Pantha rei*, the Greek aphorism meaning "everything flows, changes, or is in flux" can make a useful mantra (mantras don't have to come from Sanskrit to be effective). Sit, close your eyes and simply roll the phrase through your mind when you feel "stuck" in an unhelpful situation or relationship.

107 **Sacral chakra mantra** The *bija* mantra, or seed sound, of the sacral chakra is *VAM* (pronounced "vum"). Sitting with your spine straight, gently sing this sound to yourself to increase your ability to go with the flow when necessary.

108 **EYE AND MIRROR** *"A lake is the landscape's most beautiful and expressive feature. It is earth's eye; looking into which the beholder measures the depth of his own nature."*
HENRY DAVID THOREAU (1817–1862), USA

109 **Flow visualization** If stress drains you of the energy required to maintain equanimity, close your eyes and visualize the power of a rushing waterfall. Let its incessant flow replenish your resources and drum out tension. Whenever you have the opportunity, sit by a real waterfall, inhaling its stress-relieving negative ions.

110 **Water contemplation** As you encounter tricky situations during your day, aim to emulate the positive qualities of water, such as its readiness to yield to greater force and to flow around obstructions. Try to embody water's adaptability as well as its power to keep going despite difficulties.

111 **FLOW OF LIFE** *"When you put your hand in a flowing stream, you touch the last that has gone before and the first of what is still to come."* LEONARDO DA VINCI (1452–1519), ITALY

112 **Cupping the Void Mudra** *Dhyani Mudra* To make this contemplative gesture, sit upright and rest your palms in your lap cupped one inside the other. Then bring your thumbs together so that they barely touch. This hand position signifies emptiness, implying a state of total oneness with life's journey.

113 **GOING WITH THE FLOW** *"Make the best use of what is in your power, and take the rest as it happens."* EPICTETUS (c.55–c.135), GREECE

114   **Lightness energy lock** *Uddiyana Bandha*, or "flying up lock", is
the second of the primary yogic energy locks. Applying this lock
helps to develop a lightness and fluidity both in movement and
in thoughts by removing sluggishness in and around the sacral
chakra (see p17). To practise, subtly lift your abdominal muscles
inward and upward, toward your spine. It can help to think of the
action as engaging a muscular "energy belt" around your lower
abdomen. Once you have become familiar with the sensation,
practise it both as you move into and hold asanas. It will help not
only to build more intelligent body alignment, but also to protect
your back and tone your stomach muscles.

115   **Fluid from the core** Aim to initiate every movement today from
your body's centre of gravity, the area between your navel and
pelvis. This will bring a fluid ease and grace to your movements.

116   **Mind like water** Don't rush decisions unnecessarily.
Give yourself time to mull them over, allowing
insight to bubble up to the surface from
deep within your core.

[073]

117   **Palm Tree Pose** *Tiryaki Tadasana* To bring increased fluidity to your movements, stand with your feet hip-width apart, knees slightly bent and feet well-grounded. Begin to swing your arms around your body, letting them wrap gently around you, like ribbons on a maypole. Keep your spine straight, your head tall, and twist fluidly, breathing naturally. Close your eyes and feel the sense of release throughout your body. Then relax. ➤ 127

118   **Inward practice** If the morning's events cause you to become stressed or tense, forward bends, such as **Stretching the West Pose (683)**, and inversions, such as **Shoulderstand (843)**, will help to bring you back in touch with your inner self. You'll emerge better able to listen to and engage with others.

119   **OCEAN VIEWS**

"Though inland far we be,
Our Souls have sight of that immortal sea
Which brought us hither."
WILLIAM WORDSWORTH (1770–1850),
ENGLAND

ESTABLISHING POSITIVITY

120   **Set your resolve** To encourage you to tackle challenges to the best of your ability, create a *sankalpa* (a positive resolve in the present tense) and repeat it, with conviction, three times before you leave home. For example, "I achieve my goals effortlessly."

---

121   **INFINITE POSSIBILITIES**
"One can become whatever one wants to be, if one constantly contemplates on the object of desire with faith."
BHAGAVAD GITA (400–300BCE), INDIA

---

122   **Skull-shining Breath** *Kapalbhati* This breathing technique spring-cleans your head (*kapala* means "skull", *bhati* "shining"), refreshing your brain with oxygen and removing tiredness to leave you feeling vibrant. It's best to practise it in the morning on an empty stomach. Sit with your spine straight and breathe in, expanding your belly. To exhale, pump your breath out through your nose by forcefully pulling your belly toward your spine. Let the in-breath fill your lungs naturally. Repeat 10–20 breaths, if wished. It's important to learn this with a teacher first.

123 GENTLE MASTERY OF THE MIND
"Yoga means control of the contents of the mind."
PATANJALI'S *YOGA SUTRAS* (300–200BCE), INDIA

---

124 **Positive thinking** Yoga teaches that we are what we think, so if we speak or act with an unclear mind, chaos will follow, just like wild horses pulling a chariot. Before making any decisions today, take a moment or two to connect with *satya* (truth) and positivity.

125 **SEEK THE POSITIVE WITHIN** *"Go to your bosom; Knock there, and ask your heart what it doth know ..."*
WILLIAM SHAKESPEARE (1564–1616), *MEASURE FOR MEASURE*, ENGLAND

126 **Happiness mantra** We can all waste a great deal of energy on negativity – as a result of wanting objects, lifestyles or even states of mind that we simply do not have. The yogic way is to feel satisfied with what you *do* have. If you find yourself dwelling on desires, repeat the mantra, "Happiness is what happens." As simple as it sounds, this will soon help you to feel more accepting of and positive about the here and now.

HORSE POSE

Asvatasana

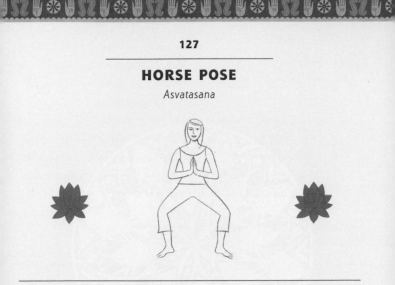

Horses (*asva*) were revered in ancient India, as recorded in the epic tale, the *Ramayana*. This positive, grounding pose recalls their balanced, noble gait.

Stand with your feet approximately 1m (3ft) apart. Turn your feet outward at a 45-degree angle, as if you were about to start a plié. Bring your palms together at the centre of your chest in **Prayer Mudra (524)** and bend your knees in line with your toes, aiming eventually to take them directly above your ankles. Breathe in positive energy. Then relax. ❯ 128

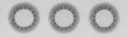

128 **Horse Pose variation** With your legs in **Horse Pose (127)**, place one palm above the other in front of your chest, as if holding an invisible soccer ball between your lower (left) palm and upper (right) palm. Inhaling, elongate your spine. Exhaling, bend to the right, feeling a stretch at the left side of your waist. As you stretch, turn the invisible ball, moving your left palm on top and your right palm beneath. Inhaling, return to centre. Exhaling, bend to the left and turn the ball again, feeling a stretch at the right side of your waist. Repeat 5 times. Then relax. ❯ 156

129 **Horse Pose vinyasa** Stand in **Horse Pose (127)** with your palms together in **Prayer Mudra (524)**. Inhaling, straighten your legs, raising your hands up through the midline of your body as you do so. Exhaling, circle your arms out to the sides and down toward the floor. Continue the flowing movement by imagining that you're scooping up stars in your upturned palms and then, without stopping, draw your palms together and up through your midline again as you inhale and straighten your legs. Continue this cycle as a *vinyasa*, or sequence of flowing movements, to bring positivity and openness to your heart area.

130 **CONTINUOUS POSITIVE MOTION** *"Put your heart, mind, intellect and soul even into your smallest acts."*
SWAMI SIVANANDA (1887–1963), INDIA

131 **Liberate your life** Freeing yourself from your individual identity brings *jivanmukti*, liberation in life, the most positive mental and emotional state you can inhabit. You achieve this precious state by identifying with the divine, spacious entity in your yoga practice, whether you call this God, Brahman, Buddha, the Tao or another name. As you hold an asana, experience the still point at the end of each out-breath, and let your mind dwell on divinity, emptiness or the creative essence of being. Other thoughts may interrupt this communion, but gently bring your attention back each time you realize that your thoughts have wandered.

132 **THIS IS YOGA**
"He is the inner Self of all, hidden like a little flame in the heart. Only by the stilled mind can he be known. Those who realize him become immortal."
SHVETASHVATARA UPANISHAD (800–400BCE), INDIA

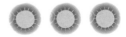

READINESS IS ALL

133   **PREPARED FOR ANYTHING** *"The readiness is all."*
WILLIAM SHAKESPEARE (1564–1616), *HAMLET*, ENGLAND

134   **Act like the Buddha** When Prince Siddharta Gautama, who later became the Buddha, set his sights upon enlightenment, he remained seated under the banyan tree in Bodhgaya, India, until he became a fully realized being. Although he was tempted from his resolve by many demons, just as all spiritual seekers are, Prince Siddharta remained rooted yet open – ready to receive transcendent awareness. In meditation, we all strive for this inner state of readiness, which prepares us for whatever life may bring each day.

135   **Enlightenment Mudra** *Bhumisparsha Mudra* This hand gesture was adopted by the "Buddha-in-waiting" as a sign of grounded openness. Sit with your spine straight. Place your left hand on your left knee, fingers pointing downward, to touch the ground. Place your right hand on your right knee, palm up like an open cup, signifying receptivity. You now embody the law of opposite forces and are ready for anything, like Prince Siddharta.

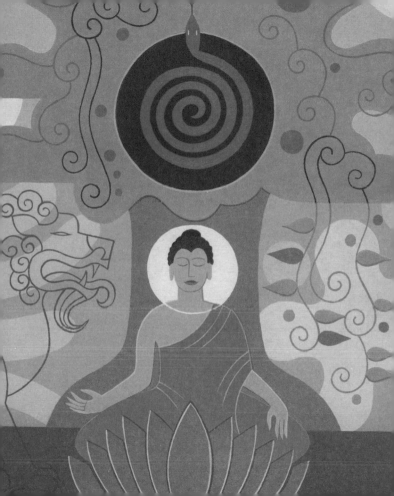

136   **Ready to learn** The term *guru* (see Sanskrit, right) means a spiritual teacher and derives from the Sanskrit words *gu*, meaning "darkness" and *ru*, "light", so a guru is someone who offers you 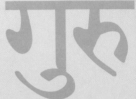 a torch in the darkness. Be attentive as you set out for the day, always looking for the *guru*, or bearer of light, in others.

137   **Morning blessing** Before leaving the house or beginning your daily yoga practice, open yourself up to what this day can bring you by repeating the following Sanskrit blessing for peace: *Loka samasta sukhino bhavantu* – "May happiness be unto the world."

138   **Ready to ride the storms** Just as there are peaks and troughs in every day, and you can't expect to be deliriously happy in everything you do, be prepared to experience a similar rhythm of ups and downs when you practise yoga. Asanas you found easy yesterday may be unexpectedly tricky today. Be patient and try to embrace whatever today may bring your way.

139   **THE VALUE OF WAITING** *"Do you have the patience to wait until the mud settles and the water is clear? Can you wait until the right action arises by itself?"*
LAO TZU (c.604–c.531BCE), CHINA

140   **The power of thoughts** Yogic philosophy states that whatever a person's mind dwells on intensely and with firm resolve, that is exactly what he becomes, so be mindful of what you spend your time thinking about and wishing for!

141   **An inner journey** Be aware that you can only put each day's external events into perspective by journeying within.
   Value yourself (142) Heed St Augustine who said: *"People travel to wonder at the height of the mountains, at the huge waves of the sea ... and they pass by themselves without wondering."*

---

143   **YOUR TIME IS NOW**
"If you desire a glorious future, transform the present. There is actually no other choice."
PATANJALI'S *YOGA SUTRAS* (300–200BCE), INDIA

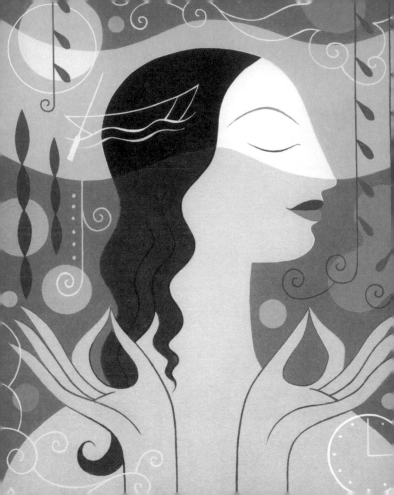

THROUGHOUT YOUR WORKING DAY

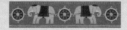

BOOSTING ENERGY

144   JUST DO IT *"Energy and persistence alter all things."*
BENJAMIN FRANKLIN (1706–1790), USA

145   Energy challenge In the *Bhagavad Gita*, Lord Krishna teaches
us that we develop the most when we have to draw from deep
within our energy reserves to meet challenges. *"Do your duty"*,
he urges, *"for action is far superior to inaction."*

146   Use it or lose it For many of us, work involves sitting at a
desk. Bodyworkers and yogis recognize that this restricts natural
movement in the lower back, hips, backs of the thighs and calves,
which prevents energy from flowing freely around the body. Re-
energize these areas by taking regular breaks to stretch your legs.

147   Crossed wires Sitting cross-legged causes postural restrictions
that halt energy flow. Avoid this by sitting with both feet flat on
the floor when possible and your spine lengthened and straight.

148   Energize your joints When your body feels weary, refresh
your shoulder joints using Head and Shoulder Rolls (see p24).

149 **Dance in your chair** Stimulating your digestive system can help to replenish vital energy when you feel that you're beginning to fade. To do this while at your desk, try some yogic seated twists: simply sit sideways on your seat, with your feet flat on the floor, and twist toward the back of the chair, placing your hands on its backrest. Take 5–10 breaths. Then return to centre, turn to face the other way on your chair and twist to the back again.

150 **Inhale energy** When you hit a mental energy slump, stretch your arms up, interlock your fingers and turn your palms to face the sky. Inhale deeply, then exhale very slowly, imagining toxins leaving your body – repeat until you feel less sluggish.

151 **Reboot your eyes** During a break from work, sit with your spine straight, close your eyes and face the sun. Allow the light to filter into your closed eyes (never look directly at the sun), then vigorously rub your hands together until hot. Place your palms over your closed eyes and imagine the warmth recharging them. Repeat 2–3 times.

152 **Save your resources** Worrying unnecessarily uses up valuable energy reserves. Follow the advice of the *Bhagavad Gita*: do your work with integrity, then rest, letting go of anxiety about results.

153 **Listen to your body** Often, when your mental energy is flagging due to over-exertion, it is a good idea to step away from your work and tune into your "body energy". Stretch up into **Raised Mountain Pose (156)** and observe your breath in and out.

154 **Turn off the world for a while** When tasks become really overwhelming, take a five- or ten-minute "energy nap", covering your eyes with an eye mask or scarf and sealing off external sounds with ear plugs to give your mind space to file away information. You'll return to work seeing everything more clearly.

155 **Revitalize your mind** The *Upanishads*, yoga's earliest Vedic texts, take their name from the Sanskrit roots *upa*, meaning "close beside", and *nishat*, meaning "to sit" – reading these writings is akin to receiving yoga teachings direct from a master. Carry a copy to dip into during breaks at work to raise your enthusiasm.

156 **Raised Mountain Pose** *Hasta Tadasana* This pose recharges body and mind by allowing energy to flow freely up and down your spine. Stand with your feet hip-width apart, fixing your gaze on a spot in front of you, then rise on to your tip-toes. Breathing steadily, raise your arms overhead, palms facing each other, and stretch through your whole body. Take 10 breaths, visualizing positive energy charging your cells. Then relax. **>** 178

157 **Energetic intentions** The intention you bring to yoga is as important and energizing as the postures themselves. In asana practice, make sure that your positive motives for practising inform every single movement so that you stretch and bend with as much positive intention as possible.

158 **CHARGING YOUR POSTURES** *"Without intention, all these postures, these breathing practices, meditations, and the like can become little more than ineffectual gestures. When animated by intention, however, the simplest movement, the briefest meditation, and the contents of one breath cycle are made potent."*
DONNA FARHI (BORN 1959), NEW ZEALAND

[089]

159   **Nature's flow** In nature, energy
builds as the moon waxes (grows)
and dissipates as it wanes (becomes
smaller). Study the moon and/or
a moon calendar over a month
to identify how your emotions
and energy tend to ebb and flow in
accordance with the moon's phases.

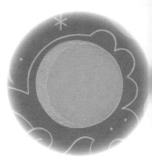

At peak energy times, tap into the moon's **Creative force
(160)**; at times of less energy, **Keep things gentle (161)**.

160   **Creative force** *Rajas*, the yogic quality, or *guna*, of ripening
equates with the energy of the waxing moon. Take advantage of
rajasic energy in your working month by initiating ideas, launching
ventures and guiding projects to fruition as the moon is growing.
In terms of yoga, this may be a time for a challenging practice.

161   **Keep things gentle** When the moon is waning, you may feel
it's best to opt for a gentle approach to both work and yoga
practice in order to nourish, rather than force, your energy levels.

162   **Right exercise** Always try to follow your instincts when it comes to your ever-changing needs and energy levels – in tune with the yogic theory of right exercise (see p23).

163   **Hold back** It is best to be cautious at full moon. Do not force work activities at this time, when both emotions and energies run high. You might prefer meditation to asana practice.

164   **Food for the brain** When you feel peckish at work or hit an afternoon slump, avoid junk food and instead snack on energizing *sattwic* foods: fresh fruit, nuts and seeds offer a brain-stimulating mix of protein, vitamins, minerals and fatty acids.

165   **Energy grazing** To keep energy high, many yogis eat little and often through the day, rather than over-eating at one mealtime.

166   **Energizing detox** Have a twice-a-year break from something unhealthy that you usually consume every day, such as sugar, alcohol or caffeine, by cutting it out of your diet for a month. *Tapas*, disciplined practice or "austerity", boosts your resources.

167 **Yoga eating** Many yogis follow a vegetarian regime. Try to include non-meat sources of protein in your diet, such as eggs, soya, nuts, pulses and seeds. As well as boosting health, this supports *ahimsa* (see Sanskrit, above), or non-violence.

अहिंसा

---

168 **ANCIENT ADVICE**
"There is no wrong in eating meats or drinking wine, but abstention ... gives many benefits."
LAWS OF MANU (1500BCE), INDIA

---

169 **A middle way** Following a middle path – neither fiercely denying life's pleasures nor completely indulging in them – is a tremendously energizing discipline. Draw inspiration by remembering that this is the path that the Buddha took.

170 **The energy to keep going** Regular yoga practice gives us the energy to stay committed to the choices we make in life and the discipline, or *tapas*, to dig deep within when we falter.

ESTABLISHING SELF-CONFIDENCE

171   **SHIFT YOUR CENTRE** *"The goal of Eastern religious practice is the same as that of Western mysticism: the shifting of the centre of gravity from the ego to the Self, from man to God. This means that the ego disappears in the self, and man is god."*
CARL JUNG (1875–1961), SWITZERLAND

172   **Develop a healthy ego** Being a yogi doesn't necessarily mean suppressing your ego. It is vital to have a strong sense of who you are and a healthy confidence in your abilities. Develop your whole self by aiming to let go of fixed notions of who you are; learn about the eight-limbed path (see pp14–15); and trust any insights you receive during your asana and meditation practice.

173   **Self-strengthening sequence** "Re-rooting" yourself to the ground to draw up "earth juice" at various points in the day helps to stabilize your sense of self and therefore your self-confidence. Do this by practising key standing poses in a dynamic way, linking the movements with your breathing. Start with **Mountain Pose (57)**, moving into **Raised Mountain Pose (156)** and then into **Chair Pose (98)**. Repeat 3 times.

174   **CONTROLLING THE EGO** *"We may discriminate a thousand times, but the sense of 'I' is bound to return again and again. You may cut down the branches of a fig tree today, but tomorrow you will see that new twigs are sprouting …. If this sense of 'I' will not leave, then let it stay on as the servant of God."*
SRI RAMAKRISHNA PARAMAHAMSA (1836–1886), INDIA

175   **Confidence practice** Standing side stretches, such as **Half Moon Pose (386)** and **Triangle Pose (534)**, and backbends, such as **Camel Pose (447)**, help to build self-esteem. They do this by grounding you and opening up your breathing muscles, which boosts your oxygen intake and encourages healthy flowing prana.

176   **Stand up for yourself** When you need an instant confidence boost, take a 5-minute break from work and practise **Mountain Pose (57)** and **Warrior Pose I (178)**.

---

177   **MASTER YOUR MIND AND BODY**
"Be a warrior and arise, great warrior arise."
BHAGAVAD GITA (400–300BCE), INDIA

WARRIOR POSE I

Virabhadrasana I

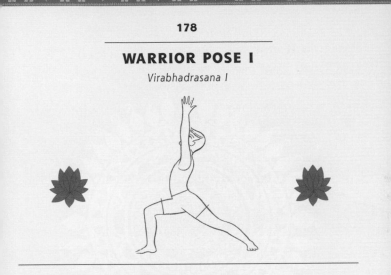

Named after warrior-sage, Virabhadra, this pose, with its sword-like arm position, celebrates the spiritual warrior within and builds self-confidence.

Stand with your feet more than 1m (3ft) apart and stretch your arms to the sides. Turn your left foot in a little and turn your right foot out by 90 degrees, rotating your legs in line with your feet.

Inhaling, lift your chest and stretch your arms above your head. Exhaling, bend your right knee until it is above your right ankle. Hold for 10 breaths, repeat to the left, then relax. ▶ 204

179 **VALUE YOURSELF** *"To be yourself in a world that is constantly trying to make you something else is the greatest accomplishment."* RALPH WALDO EMERSON (1803–1882), USA

180 **Right breathing** Yogic philosophy teaches that the way in which we breathe mirrors our innermost state. Maintaining full, spacious and relaxed breathing therefore reflects a spacious and self-assured person. Remember this during moments of self-doubt, and breathe more slowly and deeply.

---

181 **SELF-CONFIDENCE BRINGS SUCCESS** *"If you are noble, you will find the world noble."* INDIAN PROVERB

---

182 **Embrace the in-breath** Yoga teaches that the vitalizing wave of each breath is the inhalation, or *puraka*, which means "filling in". Let every inhalation root you more firmly in your strong self, and every exhalation rid you of worries and insecurities.

    Arm swings (183) To enhance the above feeling, stand in **Horse Pose (127)** and swing your arms in circles, both ways.

184 **WHO ARE YOU?**

"I am not my body
I am not my mind
I am not my emotions
Who, then, am I?"
VEDIC QUESTION

---

185 **Krama breathing** Meaning "step" or "stage", *krama* breathing
divides your inhalation into three parts, enhancing your sense
of self by slowly and gradually filling your body with fresh prana,
or life-force. Sit with your spine upright, bringing your focus to
your tail-bone. Inhale the first third of the breath from your
tail-bone to the top of your pelvis, then hold. In the second
phase of breath, try to feel your breath moving from the top
of your pelvis to the space behind your heart, and hold. Then
on the third part of the inhalation, try to sense your breath
moving from your heart to the crown of your head, and hold.
Exhale, releasing the breath in a wave from the crown of your
head to your tail-bone. Repeat 3 times. Do not hold your
breath if you feel discomfort at any stage.

186 **Feel your navel chakra** Your third, or *manipura*, chakra (see p17) – which relates to your personal power, drive and ambition – is at your navel. Focusing on its *yantra*, or visual representation (see right), helps to feed this power centre. Imagine the yellow warmth and red fieriness radiating from its ten petals, charging you with renewed energy.

187 **Self-defining mantra** The navel chakra's *bija mantra*, or seed sound, is *RAM* (pronounced "rum"). Repeat the sound silently when you need help believing in yourself or completing a task. When possible, let your eyes rest on the mantra's Sanskrit form as you chant it. This appears in the centre of the chakra's *yantra* , or visual representation (see above).

188 **Hara flame** The Japanese word *hara*, meaning "belly", describes your body's centre of self-esteem. Close your eyes and visualize a fire around your navel, energizing your entire being.

[098]

189   **Strengthen your hara** Strong standing postures, such as the
two **Warrior Poses (178)** and **(227)**, and twists, such as **Seated
Spinal Twist (737)**, bring vibrant, confident energy into the core
of the body. Make time to practise poses like these when you feel
in any way intimidated or insecure.

190   **Fire in your belly** Working the legs well in your asana practice
– or even just as you walk around during the day – increases
"fire in the belly", which promotes not only digestive efficiency,
but also the assimilation of new ideas and your zest for life.

191   **Excess fire** If you find that your sense of self has become
so strong that it begins to isolate you from others, try to see
beyond yourself and return to the ethical concepts that form
the foundation of hatha yoga practice – especially the five
yamas, or restraints, of the first limb of practice (see p14).

192   **SIMPLY BE YOURSELF** *"When you are content to be simply
yourself, And don't compete or contend, You will gain true respect."*
LAO TZU (c.604–c.531BCE), CHINA

COPING WITH STRESS

193 **THE ANSWER IS YOGA**
"Yoga is serenity."
BHAGAVAD GITA (400–300BCE), INDIA

---

194 **A sacred space** Create your own personal, distraction-free space for meditation and asana practice at home. Make it a place you can return to where you can "switch off" completely. Site it beside a window if possible so that you can reflect on nature.

195 **Make a shrine** Place a candle, flowers or an inspiring image on a low table in your sacred space as a focus for contemplation.

196 **Symbol meditation** Choose a meaningful spiritual symbol to focus or meditate upon during times of stress. A butterfly, for example, can symbolize the soul's ability to transcend difficulty, or a candle's golden light can represent positive energy.

197 **The monsoon crow** Swami Satyananda Saraswati highlights the importance of meditation symbols through the story of a crow sleeping in a tree during a monsoon storm. During the night, the tree is uprooted and floats downstream and out to sea. Waking on his floating branch, the crow sees no land. He flies East. There is no land. Then West. No land. To the South and North, there is no land either. The crow realizes that he must rest, and returns to his branch. Recovered, he again searches for land, but this time returns to his branch between flights. It becomes his resting place and reference point until he eventually finds land. In meditation – and stressful times – a symbol provides a similar anchor and resting point while you explore your mind.

198   **Soothing mantra** When you feel frazzled, sit quietly with your spine straight, and sing the *bija mantra,* or seed sound, *SOM* (pronounced "sohm") in order to soothe the nervous system.

199   **YOGIC TRANQUILLIZER** *"Today, more than at any other time in the history of humanity, people in the West are facing stresses and tensions that are beyond their control … Yoga, the oldest science of life, can teach you to bring stress under control – not only on a physical level, but on mental and spiritual levels too."*
SWAMI VISHNU DEVANANDA (1927–1993), INDIA

200   **Know your nervous system** When you feel calm, your parasympathetic nervous system is in charge, and body systems such as respiration, digestion and elimination work smoothly. When you feel stressed, your sympathetic nervous system takes over and the "fight-or-flight" response kicks in, leading to "stress" symptoms such as shallow breathing and a racing heart.

    Roll out your mat (201) Doing asanas in times of such stress encourages the parasympathetic nervous system to override the "fight-or-flight" response and restores a relaxed body and mind.

202   **Balancing stress** A certain amount of stress can strengthen your immune system, as long as it is countered with adequate rest time – self-reflection and, preferably, meditation. When you're going through a particularly stressful period, do a daily meditation to keep yourself balanced (choose from the "menu" on p375).

203   **Invaluable yoga** It is at stressful times that you most need yoga – to release tension. Yet this is the toughest time to make yourself practise. Rest assured that you're not alone in finding it hard to get motivated, so coax yourself into a ten-minute session.

WIDE-LEGGED STANDING FORWARD BEND

Prasarita Padottanasana

This semi-inverted pose boosts circulation to the upper body and brain, soothing the nervous system and easing stress. It offers the opportunity to explore the harmonious, clear-headed quality of *sattwa* (balanced energy).

When you next feel really frayed, find a quiet space and stand with your feet 1m (3ft) apart and parallel to each other. Take a deep in-breath, lifting your chest. Exhaling, fold into a forward bend and place your hands on the floor on either side of your head. Release your neck to allow your head to drop. Hold for 10 breaths. Come up slowly. Then relax. > 227

205 LET YOGA HELP

"Yoga is the destroyer of pain."
BHAGAVAD GITA (400–300BCE), INDIA

---

206 Ganesh Mudra The Hindu elephant god Ganesh has the power
to disperse both material and spiritual obstacles. Many yogis
appeal to him to resolve problems, whether at work or at home.
To ask for help, place the back of your left hand in front of your
heart with your fingers crooked. Place your right hand in front of
your left, palm facing your heart, slotting
its crooked fingers into your left hand.
Exhaling, pull your hands apart
strongly, with a chain-like grip
that creates tension in your
chest and arms. Inhale and
release the tension. Repeat 6
times. Then put your hands on
your chest to sense any new
feelings of inner strength.
Swap hands and repeat.

207 **Recognize your stress cycles** Yogis believe that everything in nature – including us – moves in cycles. When your body is in a stressed phase, don't strive for peak condition – this leads to even more stress. Avoid strenuous asanas and do more meditation.

208 **Tension-release exercise** If you feel uptight, lie on your back in a quiet place for five minutes. Inhaling, flex your feet, tighten your thighs and tense your buttocks. Let go as you exhale. Then inhale and tense your arms and hands, lifting your shoulders toward your ears. Let go as you exhale. Next, inhale and tighten your abdomen and chest. Let go as you exhale. Finally, tense your entire body, including your face, and hold your breath. Exhale as if deflating a balloon before rolling over, getting up slowly and drinking a glass of water.

209 **Store within** As you sit or lie in relaxation after the **Tension-release exercise (208)**, close your eyes and guide your mind back to a special time – perhaps a cherished summer holiday. Bathe in the comforting feelings that the memories evoke and store this energy to draw upon when you need sustenance.

210 **Mirror of the mind** The sage Patanjali suggests that the way we breathe, if erratic, is the root cause of psychological disharmony.

Slow, deep breathing (211) Good breathing is of paramount importance to good health, so remember, in times of stress, to observe your breathing reminding yourself to keep each breath even and long. This will bring you into the present moment, where you are free from stress of the past or the future.

212 **Rebalancing breath** To calm your nervous system and soothe a stressed mind, sit comfortably with your hands in *Jnana Mudra*: tips of your thumbs and index fingers touching **(96)**. Then practise **Alternate Nostril Breathing (69)**. Take 12 breaths (6 on each side). Do you feel a renewed sense of calm?

213 **Pace yourself** Go slowly at stressful times: rather than spending your commuter journey working, submerge yourself in a book.

214 **LIVE SLOWLY** *"All mankind's troubles are caused by one single thing, which is their inability to sit quietly in a room."*
BLAISE PASCAL (1623–1662), FRANCE

215 **Learn from the tortoise** In Aesop's fable *The Hare and the Tortoise*, the hare rushes ahead, but his mind is scattered and, like a stressed worker, he forgets the matter in hand. The tortoise calmly and methodically walks the path, arriving at his destination before the hare – and with energy to spare! The tortoise symbolizes the merits of looking inward and pacing yourself at times of stress. Take a leaf out of his book.

216 **A WAY OF LIVING**
"Yoga is the supreme secret of life."
BHAGAVAD GITA (400–300BCE), INDIA

217 **Value introspection** To survive a stressful day, it's important to create time for yourself to draw inward with *pratyahara*, or sense withdrawal – the fifth of the eight limbs of yoga (see p15). Encourage this by practising forward bends such as **Stretching the West Pose (683)**. It will make you feel more relaxed.

INCREASING MOTIVATION

218   **What's driving you?** When your motivation is fading, ask yourself in a quiet moment what inspires you to get up in the morning, to work, to relate to others? Yoga urges us to keep questioning and tapping into our innate driving force.

219   **CONTINUAL EXPLORATION**
"For whom are you walking?"
NATIVE AMERICAN SAYING

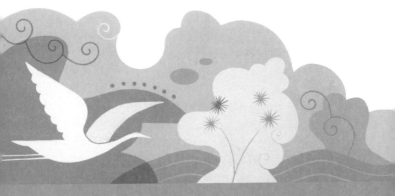

220   **Motivation visualization** When you're feeling particularly demotivated or lethargic, sit quietly with your eyes closed and picture a coiled snake with her tail in her mouth. This symbolizes the never-ending circuit of your innate, motivating energy – known as *kundalini* – which is often depicted as sleeping at the base of your spine. Practising yoga asanas, pranayama, mantras and meditation with commitment is the key to unlocking this dormant potency.

221   **YOUR DIVINE MOTIVATION** *"It is through your body that you realize you are a spark of divinity."*

B.K.S. IYENGAR (BORN 1918), INDIA

222   **Find the source within** Whether we know it or not, yoga makes us aware of our hidden human motivation: to return to the source of all life by igniting a divine spark deep within us. The *Upanishads* use the image of a swan to describe the soul's yearning for this mystical unknown. Flying over the ocean in search of herself, she finally comes to realize that "God" has been nearby all along, within herself.

223 **Trust in a greater force** All too often, we are so busy obsessing about our own motivations and desires, that we neglect the needs and desires of those around us. When you next feel wrapped up in your own worries, try to place your trust in a greater force. This will free up more time and energy for you to devote to others.

224 **Expect surprises** Is your door open to sources of inspiration from unexpected directions, beyond your everyday experience? Yogis get used to seeing the world upside down and back to front in their asana practice. Try to maintain this fresh way of seeing the world when back on two feet.

225 **JUST DO IT** *"Be daring, be fearless and don't be afraid that somebody is going to criticize you or laugh at you. If your ego is not involved, no one can hurt you."*
MAHALA PUNATEER (BORN 1965), INDIA

226 **Warrior thinking** To imbue yourself with the motivation of a noble warrior when you feel the need, repeat this affirmation: "I am strong. I am centred. I achieve my goals."

WARRIOR POSE II

Virabhadrasana II

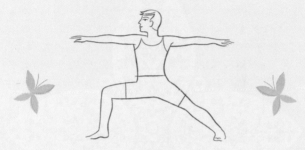

The fearless warrior Virabhadra, for whom this pose is named, was said to have defeated his enemies with a thousand arms. Channel his strength and determination in this Warrior Pose variation.

Stand with your feet more than 1m (3ft) apart, arms out to the sides. Turn your left foot in slightly and your right foot out by 90 degrees. Inhale and then exhale, bending your right leg to a 90-degree angle, with your knee above your ankle. Keep equal weight on both feet. Take 10 deep breaths. Then straighten your right leg to repeat on the other side. Then relax. > 235

228 **Give yourself** *Karma* literally means "action" (see Sanskrit, right), so *karma yoga* is a path of selfless action that regards work as a spiritual practice. To tap into this approach, give yourself wholeheartedly to a task or to your job.

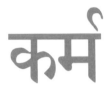

229 **YOUR CALL** *"Do what you can, with what you have, where you are."*
THEODORE ROOSEVELT (1858–1919), USA

230 **Work without grasping** Yoga teaches us to maintain a steady resolve at work. We arrive at this by detaching our emotions and motives from end results, focusing instead on the process.

---

231 **DETACHED MOTIVATION**
"Yoga is equanimity in success and failure."
BHAGAVAD GITA (400–300BCE), INDIA

---

232 **Make someone laugh** If you have an excess of motivation, you may adopt a relentless approach to work. Bringing some levity to the workplace takes the pressure off everyone and shows that you're following the middle way advocated by the Buddha.

233   **A LIGHT HEART MOVES YOU** *"Feeling light within, I walk."*
NATIVE AMERICAN SAYING

234   **Zestful energy** Asanas and pranayama seek to rebalance the body's *pran vayu*, or vital zest, which resides in the chest. This is one of five forms of prana in the body.

235   **Supported backbend** To increase *pran vayu*, or vital zest, and to boost motivation, place a soft bolster on the floor and lie back on it so that your upper spine bends over the support. Relax, breathing smoothly, for 5 minutes, enjoying an opening stretch in your chest and a lift around your heart region. **>** 250

236   **Boost your conviction** Backbending can feel exposing at first, since it opens your chest. To overcome these worries, repeat a *sankalpa*, or positive affirmation in the present tense, as you hold the pose. For example, " I meet every occasion without fear."

237   **A LIFE'S WORK** *"Your work is to discover your world and then with all your heart to give yourself to it."*
THE BUDDHA (c.563–c.483BCE), INDIA

238   **Light yourself up** In moments of self-doubt, close your eyes and visualize light infusing the cells of your body as you inhale. Let it strengthen your resolve and ignite your motivating force.

239   **Drink in oxygen** If city living wears away your zest for life, get into a green space regularly to do pranayama techniques (choose from the "menu" on p375). Fresh air boosts get-up-and-go.

240   **Seek a fresh viewpoint** When you next need fresh insight, try lying on the ground and looking up at the sky, raising your legs against a tree to get a different perspective on the world. Alternatively, practise **Shoulderstand (843)**.

241   **A NEW PERSPECTIVE** *"You must be the change you wish to see in the world."*
MAHATMA GANDHI (1869–1948), INDIA

MAINTAINING FOCUS

242 **Balance to focus** All balancing postures cultivate concentration, whether balancing on one leg, as in **Eagle Pose (321)**, on your arms, as in **Crane Pose (415)**, or simply learning to stand well on your own two feet in **Mountain Pose (57)**. If you're steady on your feet, you are more likely to maintain a focused mind.

243 **Meditate in a balance** To hold a balance such as **Dancer Pose (283)** with poise and focus, try simply to "be" in the moment: do nothing but watch your breathing.

244 **FOCUSED THOUGHTS, FOCUSED BODY** *"Thought is the sculptor who can create the person we want to be."*
HENRY DAVID THOREAU (1817–1862), USA

245 **Infinity gaze** To increase focus at work or in asanas, fix your gaze on a still point in front of you. Soften your eyes so that your gaze (or view, or *drishti*) becomes meditative and liquid: this is called "infinity gaze".

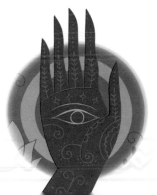

246   SELF-BALANCE
"Yoga is constancy and equilibrium –
a place that is ever the same."
BHAGAVAD GITA (400–300BCE), INDIA

247   Stand firm When you're feeling a lack of focus at work, think about the stabilizing qualities transmitted by standing asanas. Imagining yourself in one of the **Warrior Poses – (178)** or **(227)** – will help to restore a focus to get you through the day.

248   STAY ON YOUR PATH *"Pursuing the task of everyday life, I walk along the ancient path. I am not disheartened in the mindless void."* CHIKAN ZENJI (9TH CENTURY CE), CHINA

249   Give the mind space Take a break now and then to practise a standing balance pose such as **Tree Pose (250)**. Fix your eyes on a still point in front of you. Then widen your focus slightly and notice how this broadens your thinking. Observe whether this causes any original ideas to spring forth and, if so, take them back into your working day.

TREE POSE

Vriksasana

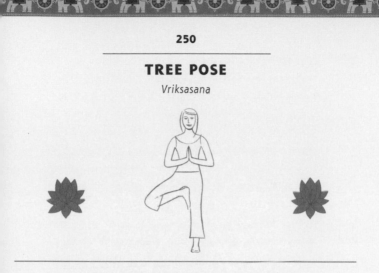

Vriksa means tree in Sanskrit, and in this pose
you emulate the steady balance and vertical focus of a tree,
firmly rooted in the earth yet growing up toward the sun.

Stand with your feet facing forward. Lift one foot and rest the sole on the inner thigh (or below the knee) of your standing leg, opening your hip. Lift your chest, anchor your tail-bone and lengthen your spine. Bring your palms together in **Prayer Mudra (524)**. Take 5 deep breaths. If you can, stretch your arms above your head. Repeat on the other side, then relax. ➤ 283

251 **Sharpening your gaze** Sit with your spine straight in a place where you see the horizon or have a good view. First, focus your eyes on the tip of your nose, then switch your focus to the horizon line or the furthest point you can see. Refocus on your nose, and then on the distant point. Repeat this shift in gaze as often as possible (stopping if it causes any discomfort). Then close your eyes. This practice strengthens your eye muscles by changing the focal length of the eyes' lenses.

252 **Pure concentration** Pay attention to *dharana*, or concentration, the sixth limb of yoga (see p15), by practising exercises that focus your mind on a still point, such as **Candle Gazing (254)**. Concentration leads your mind quite naturally into meditation, and from there into the balanced mind-state of *samadhi*, or bliss.

253 **ABSORBED IN ONE OBJECT** *"The mind generally takes up various objects, runs into all sorts of things. This is the lower state. There is the higher state of the mind, when it takes up one object and excludes all others."*
SWAMI VIVEKANANDA (1863–1902), INDIA

254   **Candle Gazing** *Tratak* This exercise uses an object of focus to still the mind, deepening yoga practice and helping you to maintain concentration. Sit in a quiet place about 1m (3ft) in front of a lit candle. Straighten your spine and be mindful of your breathing, then concentrate on the flame, gazing intently at it until your eyes begin to water slightly. Then close your eyes and visualize the flame in your mind's eye for two minutes to develop inner focus. Open your eyes ever so slightly, becoming aware of a simultaneous inner and outer focus. Finally, open your eyes fully.

255   **INNER VISION** *"Who looks outside, dreams.*
Who looks inside, awakens."
CARL JUNG (1875–1961), SWITZERLAND

256   **Soothe your eyes** After a yoga concentration exercise such as **Candle Gazing (254)** or a long period of looking at a computer monitor, warm your palms by rubbing them briskly, then place them over your eyes and look deep into your "mind cave" to rest your eyes.

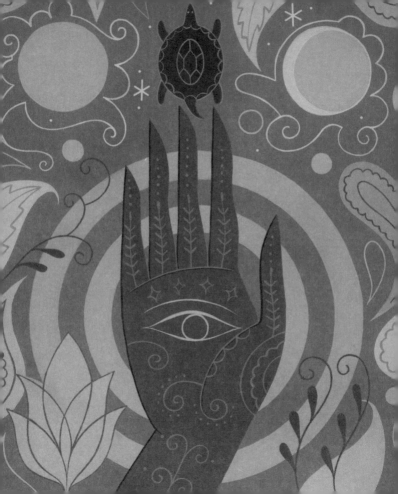

257   **THE EYE OF THE HEART** *"There is a road from the eye to the heart that does not go through the intellect."*
G.K. CHESTERTON (1074–1936), ENGLAND

258   **Inner focus** Your sixth chakra, *ajna* chakra (see p18), is your site of inner seeing (a potential source of extra-sensory perception). Known as the "third eye", this intuitive energy centre is linked by yogis to the pineal gland in the brain, which is understood to be the place from which the hormone melatonin is secreted, helping to regulate the body's natural energetic rhythms. To focus your "yogic" eye and promote the production of melatonin, it is a good idea to meditate regularly upon this chakra by gazing at its *yantra*, or visual representation **(973)**. Yogis perceive that stimulating the chakra with this sort of meditation can help to sustain you through a long day, especially if your sleep patterns have been disturbed by late nights, insomnia or jetlag.

259   **CLEANSED SIGHT** *"If the doors of perception were cleansed, everything would appear to man as it is, infinite."*
WILLIAM BLAKE (1757–1827), ENGLAND

260 **HONE YOUR SIXTH SENSE** *"It's not what you look at that matters, it's what you see."*

HENRY DAVID THOREAU (1817–1862), USA

261 **Refocus your inner eye** At work, use your inner eye of discernment to focus on information that will nourish you and to censor information that will not. Being distracted by senseless gossip at the water-cooler, for example, can focus your thoughts into unhelpful *samskaras* or "mind grooves", such as judging, which hinder personal growth.

262 **Look nearer home** *Sangham* means "coming together" and is about finding community. Sharpen your focus to block out the world of TV trivia and wake up to what is happening on your own street. Why not think about what you can contribute?

263 **A new lens** If your focus is disturbed by negative people in your workplace or by negative thoughts in your own head, retreat from your work station for 10 minutes to practise the cleansing **Lion Pose (27)** 5 times.

264   **Focused relaxation** Yoga relaxation is not the same as falling asleep! The idea is to become so still and focused that you feel revitalized afterward, ready to return to work newly focused. Try to relax in this way for ten minutes a day. It may help to listen to peaceful music. Alternatively, just stay silent – the most effective practice of all, according to the *Vedas*.

265   **Relaxation tools** It can be helpful to create your own set of relaxation tools if you find it hard to switch off. For example, you might decide to (1) tune into the rhythm of your breath; (2) scan for *samskaras*, negative ways of thinking that disrupt your focus; (3) think up and repeat a positive statement that addresses these.

266   **Potter about** Enjoy some unfocused time as you tidy your desk or a drawer, and respect any impulses that surface as you do this. Yogis view these impulses as opportunities for inner illumination.

267   **Playful focus** When meditating, gently focus your scattered mind through relaxed awareness: simply be aware of your mind at play rather than forcefully suppressing thoughts that come up.

CLEAR COMMUNICATION

268   **SWEET WORDS** *"Only speak the truth that is sweet."*
SRI K. PATTABHI JOIS (BORN 1915), INDIA

269   **Every word counts** Yogis try not to waste words, but, rather, to draw on the truth within (*satya*) before speaking.

270   **FIRST THINK** *"Before you speak, ask yourself, is it kind, is it necessary, is it true, does it improve on the silence?"*
SRI SATHYA SAI BABA (BORN 1926), INDIA

271   **Meditate to communicate** Speaking from the heart requires courage and clarity, qualities associated with the chakras above and below the heart (the throat and navel, see pp16–18). To hone your communication skills, sit quietly, close your eyes and simply take your focus first to your throat and then to your navel region.

272   **Navigate the ocean within** Think of meditation as a boat by which you can journey within to find opinions worthy of communication. Without this vehicle, you may stumble along the foreshore, or wade out into ever-deepening water.

273 **Lotus Mudra** This gesture, which creates the shape of a lotus flower in front of your heart chakra, encourages communication from the heart. Place your hands in front of your heart, with the heels of your hands, your thumbs and your little fingers touching. Spread your other fingers like outstretched petals. Take 4 deep breaths, then close the flower into a bud by closing your fingers.

274 **Lotus Mudra counterpose** This hand gesture can be useful to do after the **Lotus Mudra (273)** to give a sense of rooting your thoughts before expressing them. Close both your hands into a single "bud" and then turn them to press their backs together, pointing your fingers toward the earth, like the deep roots of a lotus flower. Make sure that your forearms stay parallel to the floor and that you feel a stretch along the backs of your wrists. Repeat several times before any important meetings to help you to make your point more clearly.

275 **The dance of communication** The Hindu god Shiva communicates by dancing out the rhythms of the universe. He stands fearless amid the circle of creative forces: generation, organization and destruction. He has slain the tiger of ambition, tamed the serpent of passion and crushed the goblin of ego.

276 **Explore Indian dance** The tradition of *Bharatnatyam*, Indian classical dance, is inspired by the creative dance of the god Shiva. To explore this ancient art of communication, look out for Indian dance lessons or performances in your local area.

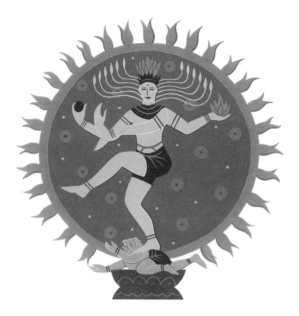

277   **Shiva inspiration** The Hindu god Shiva is an inspiration not only
for yoga and Indian dance, but also for sculpture. Buy a small
figure of Shiva in his role as Nataraja, cosmic dancer (in the pose
shown above), and place it where you need most help with your
communication skills, perhaps on your desk or by the telephone.
Let it encourage you to dance your way through life's challenges.

278 **THE POWER OF LISTENING** *"We have two ears and one mouth so that we can listen twice as much as we speak."*
EPICTETUS (c.55–c.135), GREECE

279 **Learning to hear** Press your metaphorical pause button when listening to others to really absorb what they have to say. Aim to apply this positive skill in meetings at work, being wary not to interrupt others either to control or to terminate a conversation.

280 **Listen to your body** When moving through your yoga asanas, imagine that your body can speak to you. What is it saying? Can you learn from it? Tune into this self-dialogue any time you feel a need to access the innate wisdom of your body.

281 **BE QUIET** *"He who knows does not speak, he who speaks does not know."*
LAO TZU (c.604–c.531BCE), CHINA

282 **Silent talk** Wear something at work that expresses your personality, even if only bright socks or a patterned jacket lining.

DANCER POSE

Natarajasana

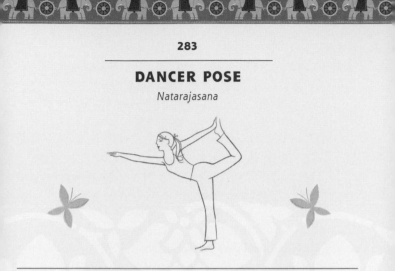

Nataraja means "King of the Dancers" in Sanskrit, and this pose helps you to use grace and poise rather than speech to communicate ideas.

Stand in **Mountain Pose (57)**, breathing smoothly and deeply. Fix your eyes on a spot in front of you, keeping your gaze soft. Lift your left foot up behind you and catch it with your left hand. Make sure you keep your hips squared. Raise your right arm in front of you, parallel to the floor. Gently arch your spine, raise your left leg behind you, open your chest and take 10 breaths. Release, repeat on the right, then relax. ▶ 302

284 **Listening meditation** *Antar Mouna* This exercise heightens your sense of hearing. Sit upright or lie on your back, and close your eyes. Tune into the sounds around you. First, choose a sound far away. Isolate it in your mind and listen to it for a while. Next, do the same with a sound near you, and then with one in the middle distance. Finally, relax and let all the sounds wash over you, without being distracted by any single one. Open your eyes and slowly resume your normal activities, with an increased awareness of all the sounds around you.

285 **Breath-sound** If you tend to get distracted when your workspace is busy, close your eyes and focus on the sound of your breathing. Listen to the waves of your inhalations and exhalations washing through you, refreshing your sense of hearing and your ability to concentrate.

286 **Communicate directly** Messages passed from person to person tend to become distorted into "Chinese whispers". Avoid second-hand information, preferring instead both to deliver and to receive messages directly.

287   **SPIRITUAL REFRESHMENT** *"So she poured out the liquid music of her voice to quench the thirst of his spirit."*

NATHANIEL HAWTHORNE (1804–1864), USA

288   **Sing it out** Limber your "communication muscles" before giving a presentation or speech by humming or singing. Let the vibrations nurture your vocal chords. You could even make up your own lyrics to express the truth you feel – *satya*.

289   **SPEAK TO GIVE** *"Communication is an offering."*

THE BUDDHA (c.563–c.483BCE), INDIA

290   **Throat-purifying mantra** *HAM* (pronounced "hum") is the *bija mantra* or seed sound associated with the throat chakra, which governs communication (see p18). Before meetings, sing the sound several times, allowing the vibrations to fortify you.

291   **Throat wash** To gain the confidence to speak honestly, sit tall, close your eyes and imagine your throat as a pillar of jade being gently "washed", or purified, by turquoise light.

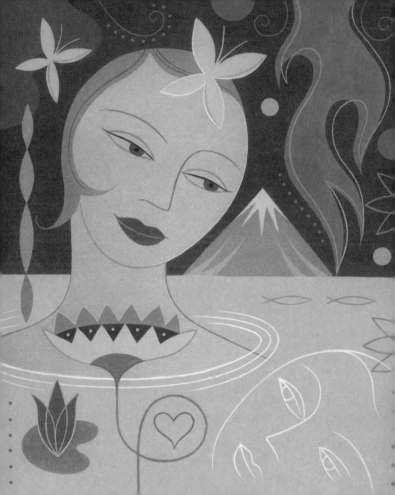

TIME FOR YOURSELF

TURNING INWARD

292 **Value introspection** Since ancient times, yogis have chosen to turn away from the sensory stimulation of the outside world to focus within. The *Upanishads* teach that when we journey inside to explore ourselves, we emerge more secure and self-confident.

293 **YOUR CHOICE**
"One path leads outward and the other inward. You can walk the way outward that leads to pleasure or the way inward that leads to grace."
KATHA UPANISHAD (800–400BCE), INDIA

294 **The true you within** *Pratyahara* forms the fifth of the eight limbs, or observances, of hatha yoga (see p15). Meaning "sense withdrawal", this inward-focused practice involves shutting out external distractions, allowing you to get more in touch with your inner self.

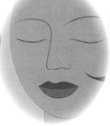

Look inside (295) A simple way to start exploring *pratyahara* is to find a quiet, comfortable space and to sit with your eyes closed for 5 minutes now and again.

296 **Tuning-in mudra** *Sanmukhi Mudra* Also known as "healthy face", this sense-withdrawal mudra offers you a quiet, soothing space within yourself when you most need it. Sit upright and place your index fingers on your eyebrows; your middle fingers on your eye-lids, closing your eyes; your ring fingers on the corners of your nostrils; and your little fingers at the corners of your mouth. Then, close the flaps of your ears with your thumbs. Rest like this for up to 30 breaths, then relax. (Avoid if you suffer from depression.)

297 **Protective poses** If you feel vulnerable after *pratyahara* practices such as **Tuning-in mudra (296)**, practise seated forward bends such as **Head-to-knee Pose (480)** or **Stretching the West Pose (683)** for the sense of security that they create.

298 **Mind-cave focus** This exercise helps you to find refuge from the outside world. Close your eyes and focus on the expansive space behind your third eye, toward the back of your skull. Also look into the space in front of your closed eyes, the *citta kash*, or "cave of the mind". Be prepared for images to appear, demanding attention, but let them pass. Open your eyes after a few minutes.

299 **Bending inward** Forward bends such as **Wide-legged Standing Forward Bend (204)** and **Intense Pose (302)** encourage *pratyahara* (sense-withdrawal) by "closing down" the front of the body (where the sense organs lie) to sensory stimulation. Taking your head lower than your heart brings fresh blood to your brain and helps thinking to become less muddled.

300 **STICK WITH IT**
"Constant practice alone is the secret of success."
HATHA YOGA PRADIPIKA (15TH CENTURY), INDIA

301 **Take it easy** Forward bends can be challenging because they stretch the back of the body intensely, which can encourage an over-ambitious, aggressive attitude. It is therefore more important than ever when doing asanas such as **Intense Pose (302)** that you maintain an approach of *ahimsa*, or "non-violence", toward yourself; forcing yourself in any way would only threaten to disrupt your sense-withdrawal practice. Be gentle with yourself by softening your knees and shoulders, and by following your breath away from the outside world, toward silence.

INTENSE POSE

Uttanasana

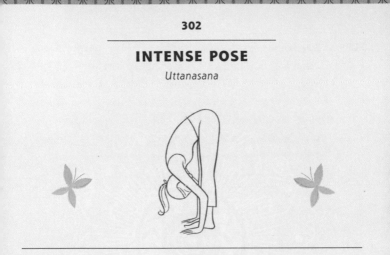

Ut means intense in Sanskrit, *tan* means to extend. By folding at the hips in this pose, your body bends in on itself for a powerful, introverted stretch.

Stand with your feet hip-width apart and lengthen your spine. Inhaling, place your hands on your hips. Exhaling, fold forward from the crease at your hips, taking your belly toward your thighs. Don't round your upper back; if you feel uncomfortable then "microbend" your knees. Aim to rest your palms on the floor at either side of your feet. Take 10 breaths, releasing tension in your neck. Gently round your spine to come back up. Then relax. ➤ 321

303 **Listening-tongue contemplation** The tongue is considered by yogis to be the floor of the brain, so by keeping silence, or a "listening tongue", you withdraw your mind from the outside world. To try this out, sit in a quiet place and rest your tongue on the floor of your mouth. Then simply "tune in" to the silence. What is it saying to you? The ancient Vedic texts state that silence brings *shanti*, or peace (see Sanskrit, right).

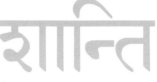

304 **YOUR MISSION** *"Only one task to do here: find out who you are. How do you find out who you are? Dive into silence and see."*
SATGURU SIVA YOGASWAMI (1872–1964), INDIA

305 **Inner-calm mantra** If you find it difficult during yoga practice to switch off from the sounds of the outside world, take your focus to your heart. When you feel ready, sing the sound *SOM* (pronounced "sohm") – the *bija mantra*, or seed sound, that calms the mind – until it resonates in your heart and quietness develops.

306   **Mind-anchor** It is natural to become distracted at first when trying to quiet the mind. It can help to have a reassuring symbol to which you can return your mind in such moments of hesitation. You might visualize, for example, a vibrant candle flame. Treat this object of concentration as a steadying "rock" if you feel lost or distracted.

307   **Become like a child** When you feel overwhelmed by the world and need some self-nurturing, drop into **Child's Pose (864)** – a deeply comforting asana that replicates the primary embryonic curve. Relax here for a few deep, even breaths.

308   **Write your own poetry** After each yoga practice, jot down any thoughts that emerge. You may like to try expressing them in poetry or creative writing as a record of your inward journey.

---

309   **DIVING IN**
"If you can give up all thoughts, you will right here and now attain the realization of oneness with all."
RAMAYANA (500–100BCE), INDIA

310 **Turning toward peace** When you make an effort on a regular basis to turn your senses away from the onslaught of the outside world, you'll gradually see just how peaceful your mind can become, as the many distracted thoughts start to quiet down.

---

311 **INNER VISION**
"Who sees the self becomes the Self."
KATHA UPANISHAD (800–400BCE), INDIA

---

312 **Beyond space and time** Regular *pratyahara* practice will lead you into *dharana*, or concentration (the sixth limb on yoga's eight-runged ladder, see p15), and then to an experience of *dhyana*, or meditation (the seventh limb), until eventually your mind dissolves in what yogis refer to as "oceanic awareness". This is *samadhi*, the eighth limb and the ultimate awakened state.

313 **Spiritual awakening** All the great religious traditions recommend times of retreat in solitude as a way of awakening the spirit. Jesus set an example by spending forty days in the desert, while the Buddha sat patiently beneath the banyan tree in meditation, ready to become enlightened. You don't have to retreat to a desert or far-off place yourself, however: your form of retreat might be to simply sit for an hour in a temple, garden or church, or to turn off the TV and sit in silence.

314 **QUENCHING SPIRITUAL THIRST** *"When he who thirsteth in the desert is silent, lo, he finds the well."*
EGYPTIAN PRAYER (c.1200BCE)

315 **Silent retreat** As you retreat from the world, look within your heart for what yogis call a "divine flame" – the spark that motivates you in life. You might contemplate the Buddha's words, *"Look within, thou art the Buddha,"* or the message of Jesus, *"The kingdom of Heaven is within you."*

316 **Yoga holidays** Every now and again, you might like to go on a yoga retreat, where a teacher can help to support you on your inward yogic journey. Such a retreat would also provide you with the opportunity to share your experiences and discoveries with other like-minded people if you so desire.

[141]

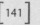

STRENGTH AND TRUST

317   **Pillars of strength** To stay strong in mind, body and emotions, make sure that you give equal attention to all five pillars of yoga recommended by Swami Sivananda – right exercise, breathing, thinking, nutrition and relaxation (see p23).

318   **Steadiness brings strength** The sage Patanjali declared that asana practice should embody *sthiram sukham*, steadiness and ease. If you establish a steady body by practising postures, a steady mind will follow suit, and you'll develop the inner strength and self-trust to meet physical and mental challenges.

319   **Strong roots** You'll derive great strength from standing poses such as **Mountain Pose (57)** and **Eagle Pose (321)**, but only if you perform them in a stable way – by "rooting" down through your inner big toe joints and outer heels before allowing your body to respond to the upward lift of your chest.

320   **THE NATURE OF STRENGTH** *"There are two ways of exerting one's strength, one is pushing down, the other is pulling up."*
BOOKER T. WASHINGTON (1856–1915), USA

EAGLE POSE
Garudasana

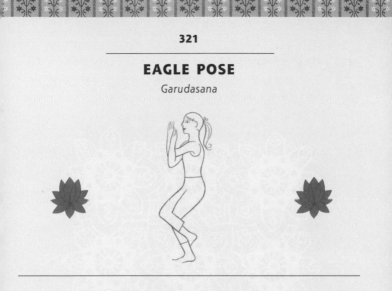

The eagle (*garuda*) symbolizes the triumph of the spirit over intellect. When you find your balance in this pose, it will bring great strength of focus.

Place your feet hip-width apart. Bend your knees and wrap your right leg around your left, aiming to hook your right foot on your left calf. Raise your arms in front, elbows bent, palms facing in. Wrap your right arm under your left and put your palms together, dropping your elbows. Hold for 10–15 breaths, with the sharp gaze of an eagle. Repeat on the other side, then relax. ➤ 337

322 THE POWER OF FOCUS

"Concentration is the secret of strength."

RALPH WALDO EMERSON (1803–1882), USA

323 Trust your instinct The *manipura* chakra (see p17), behind your navel, governs how secure you feel in your sense of self, helping to establish your level of ambition in life. To turn this navel, or "gut", centre into your personal "steering wheel", be alert throughout the day to your gut reactions and have the courage to act on them. All forms of yoga will help you to trust these instincts, increasing your sense of *satguru*, inner truth.

324 Mantra for strength If you're lacking in self-confidence, turn to the *bija mantra*, or seed sound, *RAM* (pronounced "rum"), associated with the navel chakra *manipura* – your body's power centre (see p17). Sit with your spine straight, observing your breathing. Guide your mind's eye toward your navel centre: feel your belly expanding as you inhale and contracting as you exhale. Then start to sound out the mantra *RAM*, repeating it on each out-breath until you feel stronger.

325   Food for strength Healthy eating is one of yoga's five pillars of practice (see p23). Observe how including plenty of fresh, seasonal food in your diet helps to stabilize your mood, empower your mind and therefore strengthen your moral fibre.

326   Strengthening your outer body Yogic philosophy visualizes the body as a network of five sheaths, each comprising a different density of energy (see p19). The outer sheath – the one we see – is the *annamaya kosha*, or "jacket made of food". Well-executed yoga poses are thought to strengthen this outer sheath.

327   Sun-centre visualization When you are suffering from low self-esteem, sit in **Vajrasana** (see p33) with your eyes closed. Visualize a beautiful, vibrant sunflower growing out of your *manipura* chakra, below your navel. Observe its golden hue, which echoes the powerful energy of the sun. With each inhalation, breathe in the warm, invigorating yellow energy of the sunflower until you feel its force enlivening your spirit.

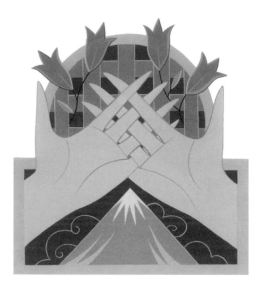

328 **Gesture of Unshakeable Trust** *Vajrapradama Mudra* In times of self-doubt, this gesture will help you to trust in your inner strength. Place your palms in front of your chest with fingers and thumbs spread wide. Interweave your fingers to create a trellis effect, then open your palms and thumbs in front of your heart. Be still, observing your breathing, for several breaths. Then relax.

329   **A strengthening resolve** To strengthen the effect of the
Gesture of Unshakeable Trust (328), repeat a powerful
sankalpa, a positive affirmation in the present tense, to yourself
silently several times while you hold the mudra. For example, you
might say, "I have great power and I channel my strength well".

330   **Empowering speech** Listen to the words you use habitually: do
you often say "must" or "should"? Boost your self-esteem by trying
to use more enabling words, such as "will" and "choose", whenever
you remember. Right speech follows right thinking (see p23).

331   **Strength and awe** *Ishwara pranidhana*, or awe in the face
of nature, is the last of the *niyamas*, Patanjali's yogic codes of
conduct (see p14). Carry with you an object that signifies the
power of nature, perhaps a special stone or a heart-shaped
talisman. Let it remind you that you are part of a wider universe.

332   **UNIVERSAL MYSTERY** *"Two things fill the mind with admiration
and awe: the starry heavens above and the moral law within."*
IMMANUEL KANT (1724–1804), GERMANY

333 **Yoga of the heart** Be inspired by people like Mother Teresa and Mahatma Gandhi, who dedicated their lives to helping others and promoting peace in the world. Such manifestations of inner strength are typical of *karma yoga* (selfless service, see p13). Strengthen your heart by doing one selfless act every day.

334 **STRENGTH OF HEART** *"The only demons in this world are those running around in our own hearts, and that is where all our battles ought to be fought."*
MAHATMA GANDHI (1869–1948), INDIA

335 **Dynamic balancing** As well as developing physical and mental strength, arm-balancing postures help you to develop a great sense of trust in yourself. Try the **Handstand preparation (337)**, then progress to **Crane Pose (415)**. Confronting fears that these poses are too difficult will strengthen your resolve.

336 **THE SECRET OF INNER STRENGTH** *"Nothing builds self-confidence and self-esteem like accomplishment."*
THOMAS CARLYLE (1795–1881), SCOTLAND/ENGLAND

337   **Handstand preparation** Only try this strengthening pose once you can comfortably maintain a diagonal line from your "outer" wrists to your hips in **Downward Dog Pose (481)**. Start in Downward Dog with your heels against a wall. Carefully walk your feet up the wall until the backs of your legs are parallel with the floor, and your arms and torso are vertical. Hold for up to 10 breaths, walk your feet down and rest on the floor. ➤ 357

338   **Emulate children** Watch how many children do handstands when playing. To become as fearless and naturally trusting as a child in such inverted poses like this, first build up your self-esteem by practising the **Sun-centre visualization (327)**.

339   **Strength of intellect** If you thrive on intellectual challenge, you may wish to look into *jnana yoga*, the path of yogic enquiry (see p13), as opposed to yogic devotion or action.

340   **Trust a greater power** Reading the yoga texts (see p11) cultivates not only intellectual strength, but a sense of awe, *ishwara pranidhana*, encouraging you to trust in a higher force.

[149]

INSPIRATION AND CREATIVITY

341   **PAINT FREELY** *"The world is but a canvas to the imagination."*
HENRY DAVID THOREAU (1817–1862), USA

342   **Connect to creativity** Yoga can be a way to connect to your creativity, because all its forms – posture practice, breathing exercises, meditations and so on – offer you glimpses beyond conditioning, deep within yourself, where anything is possible.

343   **Well springs within** Where does inspiration come from? The answer: deep within the unconscious mind. Spiritual texts often use the metaphor of fishing to describe meditative journeys into the mind – of casting a hook into the "sea of being" and then simply waiting and watching what can be drawn out.

344   **CASTING FOR INSPIRATION** *"Put out into the deep water and let down your nets for a catch."*
GOSPEL OF ST LUKE 5.4

345   **Don't snatch** It's important to practice *aparigraha*, or "non-grasping" (see p14), in all creative pursuits, including yoga.

346 **A distraction-free mind** Once you can free your mind from outward distractions through meditation, you will not only have increased access to your innate creativity but you'll also have the energy to express this in whatever way you choose. Start the distraction-filtering process by practising the calming inhalation technique, **Inspired in-breath (347)**.

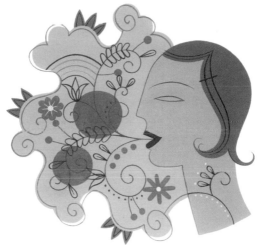

347   Inspired in-breath Each in-breath you take brings with it a
renewing and inspiring wave of energy known as *brahmana*.
Take time during your day to focus on this energy, which takes
its name from Brahman, Hindu god of creation and inspiration.

348   BREATHE IN THE SPIRIT *"Inhale, and God approaches you."*
SRI TIRUMALAI KRISHNAMACHARYA (1888–1989), INDIA

349   Inspiring backbends When you're feeling particularly
uninspired, include backbends in your posture practice to lift
your spirits. As you hold a backbend, such as **Camel Pose (447)**
or **Bridge Pose (506)**, bring your attention to each inhalation
and feel it literally re-inspiring the way you think and feel.

350   Equal breath *Asteya*, or "non-stealing", is a *yama*, advocated
by yoga's code of ethics (see p14), which you can apply to
pranayama by keeping the in- and out-breaths even: neither
"stealing" from one nor the other. Since yogis believe that the
breath mirrors the mind, this even breathing creates a calm and
balanced inner state, from which fresh ideas are more likely to

arise. Simply count to 4 as you breathe in and again to 4 as you breathe out, increasing the count as you become more practised.

351 **Making space for ideas** Exhaling makes room for the arrival of fresh prana, the life-force that flows in with your in-breath. Focus on the exhalation part of each breath when you need to make more space for free-flowing creative thought.

352 **CLEANSING BREATH** *"The out-breath … releases what is superfluous and removes what would otherwise become blocks to the free flow of prana within."*
B.K.S. IYENGAR (BORN 1918), INDIA

353 **Bellows Breath** *Bhastrika* is an invigorating practice that uses the lungs like a pair of bellows and fosters clear, creative thinking. Sit comfortably with your spine straight, breathing smoothly. Slowly draw in your breath through your nose. Then expel it in several short forceful blasts through your nose, pumping your abdomen toward your spine as you do so. Let your abdomen expand naturally as you inhale. Repeat several times if comfortable.

354 **Inner inspiration** Don't fall into the trap of trying too hard when performing asanas. A practice that is too *rajasic* (applies too much effort or zeal) will detract from your creative expression. Instead, try to let go of your attachment to the results of postures, be it a honed stomach or the desire to achieve the "final pose". This brings about a creative practice that inspires you afresh with each movement. It's also a good model for how to approach life in general: living fully in each moment.

355 **Wring out your ego** Twisting poses create a wringing-out effect that invigorates the organs, muscles and nerves, removing sluggishness and bringing about a renewing, inspiring energy. Build twists such as **Twisting Triangle Pose (357)** and **Seated Spinal Twist (737)** into every practice session.

356 **Safe twisting** To twist effectively, it's important to understand how the spine moves. The lumbar spine (lower back) is designed not to twist, but to flex forward and back. Stabilize it by engaging your core abdominal muscles, then twist your thoracic spine (back of the rib-cage) and cervical spine (back of the neck).

TWISTING TRIANGLE POSE

Parivrtta Trikonasana

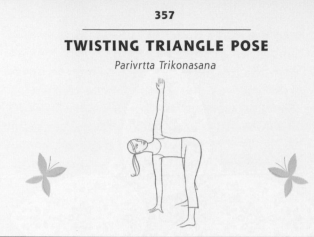

In this twisting pose, the body is at once solid, because of the grounded wide-legged stance, and fluid, due to the freeing rotation of the upper body. This balance of movement makes us open to *shakti* (creative energy).

Stand with your feet parallel, 1m (3ft) apart. Stretch your arms out to the sides. Inhaling, lift your chest; exhaling, place your right hand on the floor in front of you to create the top of a triangle shape, with your feet as its base corners. Turn your upper body left, stacking your left shoulder on top of your right. Extend your top arm. Take 5 breaths. Repeat to the right, then relax. > 386

358 **Think like a child** To foster your own creativity, spend some time with young children, watching how they play – you might like to show them how to do a fun asana, such as **Lion Pose (27)** or **Downward Dog Pose (481)**. Observe how they explore the pose without an end goal and see if you can take a little of this attitude into your own asana practice.

359 **INSIGHT THROUGH PLAY** *"Man is most nearly himself when he achieves the seriousness of a child at play."*
HERACLITUS (c.535–c.475BCE), GREECE

360 **A playful practice** Asana practice can feel like an expression of your individuality if you think of your body parts as jigsaw pieces, which can be aligned to make various puzzles: the poses. In each starting position, adopt a childlike curiosity about how you'll get to the next stage of the pose – this might not be in the conventional way. Allow your body weight and instinct free rein. By removing expectations and assumptions, you open yourself to new ways of connecting different parts of the body and fresh ways of thinking; it becomes a heart-felt practice.

361   **CREATIVE EXPLORATION** *"One must still have chaos in oneself to be able to give birth to a dancing star."*
FRIEDRICH NIETZSCHE (1844–1900), GERMANY

362   **It's not a competition** When you begin yoga classes, you may find that you display competitive tendencies, which stifle your creativity. The yogic way is to be inspired not by those around you, but by your own body and mind as they are today, which will be different from any other day and from any other yogi.

363   **Home practice** If you feel inhibited expressing yourself in yoga class, practise at home to music that touches your heart and makes you move from deep within your core. Or practise outside, letting the presence of trees, clouds and birds inspire you.

364   **A creative break** Cherish holidays, weekends and days off – the days when you step out of the clothes, roles and associations that define your working life. At these times you can recover your creative self and live life according to *satya*, your own unique and "truthful" way of being.

365   **CREATIVITY BRINGS HAPPINESS** *"To have the sense of creative activity is the great happiness and the great proof of being alive."*
MATTHEW ARNOLD (1822–1888), ENGLAND

366   **Mudra for creativity** *Agochari Mudra* This is a yogic gaze, which, accompanied by a hand gesture, soothes the nerves and concentration, boosting the potential for creativity. Sit up straight, with your hands in *Jnana Mudra*: tips of your index fingers and thumbs touching **(96)**. Focus your eyes on the tip of your nose, take several deep breaths, then relax.

367   **Yogic energy lines** Yoga philosophy teaches that our life-force, prana, travels around the body through thousands of energy lines called *nadis* (the Sanskrit root *nad* means "stream"). Asanas and pranayama techniques cleanse the nadis of energy blockages, allowing prana to travel more freely. As well as better overall health, this creates greater reserves of vibrant, creative energy.

368   **ENERGY STREAM** *"The fountains of sacred rivers flow upwards."*
EURIPIDES (480–406BCE), GREECE

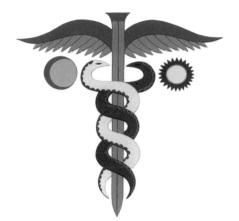

369 **Your energy channels** The caduceus (see above) symbolizes the three principal *nadis*, or subtle energy channels, in the human body. The left, or lunar, channel, *ida*, governs restorative, feminine energy, while the right, or solar, channel, *pingala*, governs active, male energy. Asanas and pranayama balance these energies, causing the latent energy, or *kundalini*, at the base of the spine to rise up the central channel (*sushumna*), freeing your creativity.

370   **CREATIVE SOURCE** *"Creativity comes from awakening and directing our higher natures, which originate in the primal depths of the universe and are appointed by Heaven."*
I CHING (c. 9TH CENTURY BCE), CHINA

371   **Adoring yoga** *Bhakti yoga*, the yogic path of worship and devotion (see p13), places emphasis on prayer, song, sacred words and meditation. If you find this surrender to a higher spiritual force inspiring, try chanting the **Mantra of Inspiring Light (372).**

372   **Mantra of Inspiring Light** *Gayatri Mantra*, one of the most sacred of all the Hindu mantras, is a song of praise to radiant light, or divine energy in feminine form. It is also a hymn to the inspiration that this divine light can bring. Singing it inspires you, protects you, awakens your intuition and illuminates your spirit. Each syllable is so loaded with potent meaning that it is best to chant it in Sanskrit, pronouncing each sound clearly and distinctly:
"Om Bhur Bhuva Swaha
Tat Savitur Vareenyam

Bhargo devasya Dhimahi
Dhiyo yo nah prachodayat."

---

373 INNER LIGHT
"Now, the light that shines above in heaven
– pervading all the spaces, everywhere, both below
and in the farthest reaches of the worlds – this is
the light that shines within a human being."
CHANDOGYA UPANISHAD (800–400BCE), INDIA

---

374 Bypass creativity blockers Being bombarded by information 24/7 can sap your creative spirit after a while. Turn off the TV whenever you can and instead read spiritually nourishing material. In yoga's eight limbs (see pp14–15), this cultivates *saucha*, "cleanliness", and *santosha*, "contentment".

375 Feed your mind well *"... intellectual poison, which takes the form of cheap newspapers or bad books, can unfortunately sometimes be attractive."*
LEO TOLSTOY (1828–1910), RUSSIA

JOY AND CELEBRATION

376   **JOYFUL ENERGY** *"The joy of a spirit is the measure of its power."*
NINON DE LENCLOS (1620–1705), FRANCE

377   **The wisdom of spontaneity** A Zen master sat down to give
a sermon just as a bird began to sing outside the room. The
master remained silent as all those present listened to the
spontaneous outburst of joyous birdsong. When the bird had
finished, the master simply smiled, pronounced the sermon
over, got up and walked out of the room.

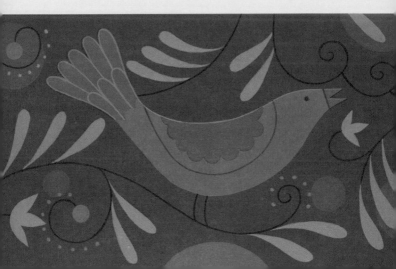

378   **Live in the moment** If you can simply "be" in the present, you will find joy in the most mundane activities. Too often the mind is distracted by the future or past, which limits your capacity to be joyfully present. All forms of yoga aim to reveal the joy of now.

379   **Embrace the present** The Buddha once said: "When you realize how perfect everything is, you will tilt your head back and laugh at the sky." Adopt this approach to life, celebrating the world and treating everything as a miracle, and each moment will feel like a precious jewel.

380   **Where joy resides** The Sanskrit term *buddhi* means "he or she who is conscious, or awake" and refers to a pure quality of mind, like that of a newborn baby. Yoga teaches that only when we replicate such a pristine awareness are we able to be fully present and spontaneously joyful.

381   **Glimpse joy** To fleetingly glimpse the joyous state of *buddhi*, find a comfortable spot outside and lie down. Look up at the sky and do nothing except observe your breath.

382   **Effortless being** Ayurveda, the ancient system of Indian healing, defines health as "bodilessness": if your body is healthy, you float through the day effortlessly – with joy. Aim to experience this lightness of being when you next practise yoga.

383   **JUST DO IT** *"... joy's soul lies in the doing."*
WILLIAM SHAKESPEARE (1564–1616), *TROILUS AND CRESSIDA*, ENGLAND

384   **Energetic poses** Asanas that make you feel light, agile and energetic cultivate joy in the wonder of the human body. Try backbends such as **Camel Pose (447)**, standing balances such as **Half Moon Pose (386)**, arm balances such as **Handstand preparation (337)** and the dynamic Sun Salutation sequence (see pp28–31). Relish the joyous energy that these poses stimulate.

385   **Inverted poses** If you feel lacking in *joie de vivre*, refresh yourself with a novel outlook on the world by doing inverted poses such as **Downward Dog Pose (481)** and **Shoulderstand (843)**. It's best to warm up first with limbering exercises and 3–5 repetitions of the Sun Salutation (see pp28–31).

HALF MOON POSE

Ardha Chandrasana

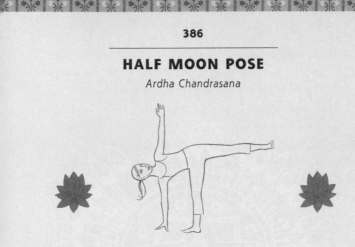

As you stretch in this pose, your body traces the smooth arc of a crescent moon (*chandra*). You will have to practise conscientiously, but when you finally balance without fear it is a feat to celebrate.

Begin with feet 1m (3ft) apart. Turn your left foot in slightly and your right foot out 90 degrees. Bend your right knee and place your right hand on the floor, or a block, by your right foot. Shift your balance to your right foot and hand, straighten your right leg, lift your left leg and extend your left arm in the air. Take a few breaths. Lower your leg, repeat to the other side, then relax. ➤ 415

387 **Twisting poses** Asanas that twist and turn the body, such as **Twisting Triangle Pose (357)**, offer a massage that squeezes out not only physical toxins, but also mental ones in the form of negative thinking, bringing about a more joyous disposition.

388 **Enjoy each pose** When you do your asana practice, take time after each posture to observe any changes in your body and state of mind. Notice which poses soothe you, which invigorate you and which cultivate joy. Then tailor your sessions to suit your changing needs.

389 **Time to breathe** It's a liberating feeling when your breath is flowing freely. Set aside time – 10 minutes if possible – at the end of each yoga session to practise breathing techniques, such as **Krama breathing (185)**.

390 **Suspended Breath** *Kumbhaka* Yogis perceive that controlled retention of the breath can bring about stillness and joy. Breathe in through your nose for 5 counts, then breathe out through your nose for 5. Repeat this several times. Then, after an exhalation, hold your breath for 5 counts, if comfortable, before inhaling. Continue in this way – in for 5, out for 5, suspend for 5 – for 1 minute. Then return to your natural breathing.

391   **Opening breath** To bring a sense of warmth and joy to your heart, take particularly slow, deep inhalations as you hold poses that gently open up the front of the body where the heart chakra is sited, such as **Bridge Pose (506)** and **Stretching the West Pose (683)**.

392   **The joy of breathing** Breathe deeply not just in yoga practice but throughout each day. Maximizing the oxygen you take in and the toxins you expel increases your zest for life at any time.

393   **Mind detox** When you're feeling low, sit quietly, close your eyes and simply observe your mind for 5 or so minutes. When any "debris" or "mental chatter" drifts into your mind – distracting thoughts or feelings – observe it without allowing yourself to connect with it. This clears your mind of clutter, making it feel lighter, and brightening your outlook.

394   **Joyous repetition** When you need a boost, inward repetition (*japa*) of a sound or phrase, can help you to feel joyous. Think up an inspiring *sankalpa*, or positive affirmation in the present tense, such as, "Joy arises within me." Repeat it silently as you go about your day until events demonstrate that it has become true.

395   **Release your mask** Brighten yourself up when you feel tired or over-worked with this "natural face-lift". Inhaling, close your eyes and screw up your face as tight as a prune. Then, exhaling, stretch out your face, feeling it light up like a radiant sunburst.

---

396   **JOY OF CREATION**
"From joy springs all creation, by joy it is sustained, toward joy it proceeds, and to joy it returns."
MUNDAKA UPANISHAD (800–400 BCE), INDIA

---

397   **Bliss mantra** We all aspire to a more blissful mental state. Chanting the Sanskrit words *Sat chit ananda* ("truth, mind, bliss") is believed to bring you toward this by dissolving *samskaras*, habitual ways of thinking and behaving that limit you.

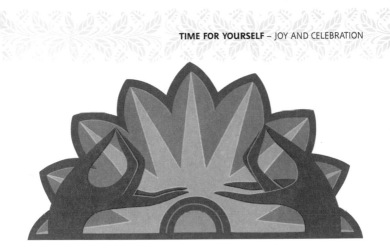

398 **Mudra for receiving joy** *Pushan Mudra* Dedicated to the Hindu sun god Pushan, this symbolic gesture fills you with the energy to give and receive joyously. On your right hand, bring the tips of your index and middle fingers to touch the tip of your right thumb. Extend your ring and little fingers. On your left hand, bring the tips of your middle and ring fingers to meet the tip of your left thumb. Stretch out your index and little fingers. Practise for 5 minutes up to 4 times a day, whenever you feel in need of a more joyous flow of energy.

FINDING BALANCE

399 **BALANCED IN UNITY**
*"Unified am I, quite undivided am I,
the whole of me."*
ATHARVA VEDA (1200BCE), INDIA

400 **The full picture** Yoga teaches that physical balance makes
us more integrated, since it allows all the body's systems to
exist in a state of harmony and to function at optimal levels.
Not only should you make sure that each asana you do feels
balanced, but also that your overall yoga practice balances
posture work with breathing and meditation.

401 **TRUE BALANCE** *"Be truly whole, and all things will return to you."*
LAO TZU (c.604–c.531BCE), CHINA

402 **Self-discovery** Spending regular quiet time with yourself in
asana and pranayama practice lets you learn more about your
own motives and discover ways to resolve issues so that your
mind becomes free of conflict. In this way, yoga moves you
toward not only physical but also mental and emotional balance.

403   **Rest and action** Imagine a pair of weighing scales. On one side is *tamas* (the force of inertia); on the other *rajas* (the force of activity). In the centre lies *sattwa* (see Sanskrit, below), a synthesis of these opposites. Aim to move toward this balanced way of being by maintaining a healthy combination of *tamas* and *rajas*, in both your asana practice and your everyday life.

सत्त्व

404   **The middle path** To work toward a state of equilibrium in your life, try scheduling some nights in if you normally have a hectic social life, or plan some down-time within a busy working day.

405   **The balance of opposites** A student told his teacher, "In order to become fully awake, we must concentrate and pray ceaselessly until we glimpse the transcendent." The master replied, "You are right." A second student said, "But we cannot fight to see what is unknown: we need to surrender, to welcome the gift of grace." "You, too, are right," said the master. A third student said, "Surely you need both; to strive to understand, and to surrender to the unknowable?" "And you, too, are right!" the master said.

406   **BALANCING THE ELEMENTS** Yogic philosophy teaches that we, like everything, are made up of earth, water, fire, air and ether. Living by Patanjali's eight-limbed path (see pp14–15) helps to balance these elements within us, leading to *santosha*, true contentment with what we have and are in life. Once we ourselves feel balanced, the world around us will also feel balanced.

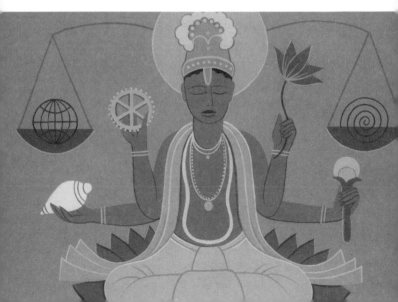

407   **ONE WORLD** *"The world will be balanced when we are balanced."*
TARTHANG TULKU (BORN 1935), TIBET

408   **Dynamic evolution** It is best to view your yoga practice as
a constant exploration – a journey toward balance. When you
approach familiar poses, think of them not as static shapes, but
as continually evolving processes that vary according to your
ever-changing physical, mental and emotional state.

409   **Zeal and surrender** The sage Patanjali advised that asana
practice should balance intensity and focus with release and
surrender. By paying attention to these opposing forces as you
move into, hold and release a pose, you not only avoid injury,
but your yoga practice becomes a form of moving meditation
– you begin to embody balance at a deeper level.

410   **All postures are balances** Consider every yoga asana
– standing, sitting, balancing, twisting and inverted poses – as
a balance. Feel how it teaches you to create a stable foundation
and to distribute your body weight evenly over that base.

411 **Begin to balance** When practising a steady posture such as **Mountain Pose (57)**, it is important to focus on distributing weight and energy equally through both feet. When adjusting your balance, think about Mountain Pose's alternative name, *sama-stithi*, which means "equal–steady".

412 **LAYING FOUNDATIONS** *"Do you wish to rise? Begin by descending. You plan a tower that will pierce the clouds? Lay first the foundation of humility."*
ST AUGUSTINE (354–430), NORTH AFRICA

413 **Working with gravity** Imagine as you do each yoga posture that the crown of your head and your sternum are fitted with anti-gravity devices that pull you upward. Then let your lower body surrender to gravity, particularly the grounding points on the soles of your feet and the joints of your big toes.

414 **Easy squat** To build up to **Crane Pose (415)**, place your feet hip-width apart and lower your pelvis into a squat. Bring your palms into **Prayer Mudra (524)** and lever your knees apart.

CRANE POSE

Bakasana

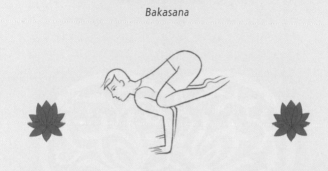

This deep arm balance evokes the elegant poise of a crane (*baka*) standing in water. Try it when you need to find your focus.

Bend your knees and place your hands on the floor between your legs, shoulder-width apart. Stretch out your fingers, then bend your elbows, making a "ledge" with your upper arms. Round your spine, engage your navel and try to rest your shins on your upper arms, guiding your knees toward your armpits. Very gradually lift your feet if you can and look ahead, balancing on your arms for several breaths. Then rest in **Child's Pose (864).** 447

416   Balance from the fulcrum The art of balancing involves positioning and keeping your fulcrum – your body's centre of gravity – above your foundation points. In standing balancing poses, such as **Tree Pose (250)** or **Dancer Pose (283)**, your fulcrum is your pelvis, and your grounding points your feet. It may help to visualize your pelvis as an immovable central point.

417   THE CENTRE *"The pointer of a pair of scales always returns to centre."*
GUSTAV MAHLER (1860–1911), AUSTRIA

418   Core balancing skills In all poses that involve balancing – whether on your feet or your hands – engage the core muscles deep in your abdomen and initiate movement from this centre.

419   "Organ-ized" balance If a standing pose is well balanced, every organ within the body's structure is given adequate space in which to function (unlike when you slouch or hunch your shoulders). To maintain this space as you twist and turn in your asana practice, think about your bones moving and visualize them creating a protective cage for your organs.

420 **INNER NORTH** *"The magnetic needle always points to the north, and hence it is that the sailing vessel does not lose her direction."*
SRI RAMAKRISHNA PARAMAHAMSA (1836–1886), INDIA

421 **Finding equanimity** Yogis seek peace that comes when we balance the layers (*koshas*) of our consciousness: body, mind, energy and emotions. Bear in mind that whether we ever arrive at our destination is unimportant; what matters is not getting lost on the way. Perhaps there *is* no fixed destination!

422 **Rebalancing time** To maintain inner balance, take time for yourself during the day. Sit somewhere peaceful for 10 minutes, following a relaxation or a meditation from the "menu" on p375.

---

423 **INWARD BALANCE**
"Let the five senses and the mind they serve become still. Let awareness itself cease all activity and become watchful. Then you have begun your journey on the highest path."
KATHA UPANISHAD (800–400BCE), INDIA

424   **Breath symmetry** Bringing your inhalation and exhalation into symmetry helps to rebalance your energies for equanimity of mind. Lie on your back somewhere comfortable and observe your navel rising and then falling each time you breathe. Aim to balance the length of each in-breath and out-breath.

425   **THE PEACE BETWEEN BREATHS** *"Complete peace equally reigns between two mental waves."*
SWAMI SIVANANDA (1887–1963), INDIA

426   **Tibetan rebalancing breath** To equalize your breathing and thereby calm your mind, sit upright and rest your hands on your thighs or knees in *Jnana Mudra* **(96)**. Take several breaths. Then, inhaling, sweep your left arm in an arcing movement up to the sky, bend your elbow, and at the peak of the inhalation, close the bridge of your left nostril with your left thumb. Smoothly exhale through your right nostril. At the end of the exhalation, rest your left hand back in *Jnana Mudra*. Repeat the movement on your right side. Work up to 6 repetitions on each side (12 breaths in total). Then relax, hopefully feeling much more balanced.

427   **Moonlight meditation** When a stream of thoughts disturbs
your inner balance, sit upright, close your eyes and imagine your
mind as a still lake at night. Picture your thoughts as ripples
gently moving across the surface of this calm, moonlit lake. When
a thought lingers as more than a ripple, disturbing the still water,
focus on the moonbeam lighting it up and trace your awareness
back to its light-source, the mystical moon. Allow its soothing
glow to seep into your being, bringing a deep sense of calm.

428   **Gesture of balance** When you feel
physically and emotionally out of sync,
place your palms together for a few
moments in **Prayer Mudra (524)**,
a gesture of inner harmony that will
bring you back into balance.

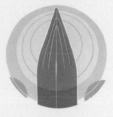

429   **BALANCED BLESSINGS** *"I offer you peace. I offer you love.
I offer you friendship. I see your beauty. I hear your need.
I feel your feelings."*
MAHATMA GANDHI (1869–1948), INDIA

[179]

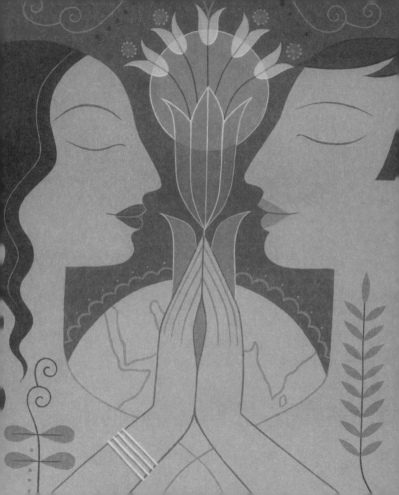

RELATING TO OTHERS

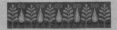

LOVE AND COMPASSION

430   LOVING WORDS
"You yourself, as much as anybody in the entire universe, deserve your love and affection."
THE BUDDHA (c.563–c.483BCE), INDIA

431   Hold up a mirror Yogic philosophy states that the soul's yearning for a connection with others derives from a yearning to connect with itself. Nourish your inner "other" by meditating daily using the exercise **Feel your heart chakra (448)**.

432   LOVE YOURSELF FIRST *"If you want a deep, intimate relationship with another, first become aware of who you are."*
WILLIAM HAUGH (1922–2007), SCOTLAND

433   Move with the breath Using your breath as a rhythmic guide when practising asanas will give your yoga more of a natural, flowing feel – which allows your emotions, too, to flow more naturally. To do this, aim with each breath either to deepen a posture or initiate a new movement.

434 **MIND-HEART UNITY** *"Regulate the breath, be happy.*
Link the mind with the Lord in your heart."
SRI TIRUMALAI KRISHNAMACHARYA (1888–1989), INDIA

435 **Create time for compassion** *Ahamkara* means "I-maker" in
Sanskrit, and represents your sense of individuality and self. If
you become too preoccupied with *ahamkara* you can become
distracted from your compassion for others, so practise the
Heart-centred affirmation (464) to avoid it dominating.

436 **Meditative treasure** Yogis perceive that the clear, uncluttered
state of mind that meditation can bring about is your deepest
potential treasure. This state of mind will unite all the scattered
parts of yourself, heightening your capacity for love and
compassion – not only toward others but also toward yourself.

437 **SELFLESSLY SERVING OTHERS** *"It is only when we want nothing*
for ourselves that we are able to see clearly into others' needs and
understand how to serve them."
MAHATMA GANDHI (1869–1948), INDIA

438 **Soften to connect** Yogic philosophy teaches that everything –
including ourselves – is made up of opposing yet complementary
forces, including masculine and feminine energy. Modern living
tends to demand that we bring our active, "masculine" energy to
the fore, as we drive ourselves at work, or in asana practice. But
this can build a protective shell that may end up isolating us.
To develop your softer side, allow your more gentle, "feminine"
aspect to surface, melting that shell. Start by trying to infuse your
yoga with a non-aggressive approach, known as *ahimsa*.

439   MELTING WITH COMPASSION *"The hardest metal yields to sufficient heat. Even so must the hardest heart melt before ... the heat of non-violence. And there is no limit to the capacity of non-violence to generate heat."*

MAHATMA GANDHI (1869–1948), INDIA

440   TAKE A LOVING APPROACH *"Practise love until you remember that you are love."*

SWAMI SAI PREMANANDA (BORN 1972), CANADA

441   Unite head and heart The spiritual leader Osho encourages us all to feel with the heart, not the head – quite a challenge in today's all too often knowledge-based, achievement-driven society. Commit yourself to feeling with your body and heart and acting on their instincts, rather than making decisions only with your brain – at first, just for one day and, then, for longer. Note how different life feels when you approach it in this way.

442   FROM THE HEART *"... the mouth of the wise man is in his heart."*

BENJAMIN FRANKLIN (1706–1790), USA

443   **Just connect** Smile at passers-by and say hello to the people you interact with in daily life. Small acts of compassion are yogic at their core and make the world a better place to live in.

444   **FOLLOW THROUGH** *"It is not enough to be compassionate. You must act also."*
TAOIST SAYING

445   **A guru's compassion** Krishnamacharya, renowned guide of yoga masters B.K.S. Iyengar, T.K.V. Desikachar and Pattabhi Jois, used to meet all his students at the gate and escort them to his yoga *shala*, or school. After class, he escorted them back to the gate. Let this mindful practice inspire you to make not only your yoga practice but also your life more connected and heartfelt.

446   **THE CHAIN OF BEING** *"The thought manifests as the word. The word manifests as the deed. The deed develops into habit. And the habit hardens into character. So watch the thought and its ways with care ... let it spring from love."*
THE BUDDHA (c.563–c.483BCE), INDIA

CAMEL POSE

Ustrasana

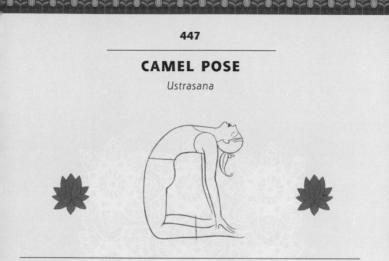

This pose is named after the camel (*ustra* in Sanskrit), because the curve of your chest, as you bend backward, resembles its characteristic hump. Bending in this way opens up your heart to love and compassion.

Kneel with your knees hip-width apart. Lift your hips and press your hands down on your buttocks, drawing your elbows toward each other behind you. Lift your chest, arch your spine and lean back to open your chest. If possible, place your hands on your heels, straighten your arms and drop your head back (see above). Take 10 deep breaths, then rest in **Child's Pose (864)**. ▶ 480

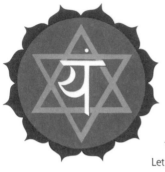

448   Feel your heart chakra
In the middle of your chest lies the energy centre where you connect with your emotions – your heart, or *anahata*, chakra. Look at its *yantra*, or visual representation (see left), and feel this as an energetic pattern in your chest. Let the heat of the 12 red petals equip you to live each moment with warmth and compassion.

449   Flame vizualisation Close your eyes and visualize a flame burning in a cave at the back of your heart. Ancient yogis called this *jyoti*, the divine spark that triggers life. Contemplating this inner light is said to fan its flame, feeding both your heart and soul (*jyoti* also means "soul").

450   Listen to your heart The Sanskrit name for the heart chakra, *anahata*, means "the centre of the unstruck sound". Do what its name urges: draw within, away from your sense organs, and tune into the pure silence of your heart.

451   **THE LOVE THAT DOES NOT SPEAK** *"My heart is so intoxicated with love that I have no wish to speak."*
KABIR (1440–1518), INDIA

452   **Backbending** When you feel the need to open your heart to get in touch with the world around you, practise backbends such as **Camel Pose (447)** and **Bridge Pose (506)**. These open your chest, heart and lungs, encouraging vitality to flow into your body and making you feel more positive and "connected".

---

453   **OPEN YOUR HEART**
"We can be spacious yet full of loving kindness; full of compassion yet serene. Live like the strings of a fine instrument – not too taut but not too loose."
THE BUDDHA, FROM THE *ANGUTTARA NIKAYA* (c.250BCE), INDIA

---

454   **Air contemplation** Contemplating the expansive nature of air, the element traditionally associated with the heart chakra, can lighten the heart: close your eyes, gaze into your heart and recognize the limitless space available for you to develop love.

455 **Heart Mudra** *Hridaya Mudra*
This hand gesture, or mudra (see
Sanskrit, right) diverts energy
flow from the hands to the heart
area, helping to address and
release pent-up emotion. Sit with your spine straight and the
backs of your hands on your thighs. Bring in your middle and
ring fingertips to meet your thumbs, keeping your index and
little fingers outstretched. Focus your breathing in your heart area.

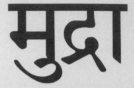

456 **YOGIC QUESTION** *"Can I see another's woe, and not be in sorrow
too? Can I see another's grief, and not seek for kind relief?"*
WILLIAM BLAKE (1757–1827), ENGLAND

457 **Metta Meditation** When you're having difficulty accepting the
actions of, or getting on well with, certain friends or colleagues,
try this healing Buddhist practice of loving-kindness. Sit with
your spine straight, close your eyes, breathe deeply and rest your
open palms on your knees in a gesture of receptivity. Firstly,
visualize yourself, then send yourself loving thoughts, repeating

to yourself, "May I be happy. May I be free from fear. May I be safe and protected." Now picture a loved one and send him or her similar positive thoughts. Next, visualize a person to whom you feel less attached and send them your love. Finally, try to send good vibes to someone you dislike or have issues with.

458 **SPREAD KINDNESS** *"Do all the good you can, By all the means you can, In all the ways you can, In every place you can, At all the times you can, To all the people you can, As long as ever you can."* JOHN WESLEY (1703–1791), ENGLAND

459 **Yoga of devotion** Bring the yoga of *bhakti*, or devotion, into your life by visiting somewhere that feels sacred to you, or by simply appreciating a remarkable piece of music or poetry. In such acts, you experience connection with everything that is.

460 **THE WAY OF WORSHIP** *"Love the animals, love the plants, love everything. If you love everything, you will perceive the divine mystery in things."* FYODOR DOSTOEVSKY (1821–1881), RUSSIA

A SENSE OF NURTURING

461 **LOOKING AFTER YOUR BODY** *"Care for your eyes and ears, then the nostrils and the tongue, the heart, stomach, navel, womb, thus every part of the body."*

SRI TIRUMALAI KRISHNAMACHARYA (1888–1989), INDIA

462 **Nourish yourself first** By bringing your own mind, body and emotions into a state of harmony, you become better able to nurture others. Think about the five pillars of yoga – right exercise, right breathing, right thinking, right nutrition and right relaxation (see p23). Do any of these need more attention in your life? If so, aim to make changes that will bring this about. You might, for example, buy more fresh fruit in your weekly shop, do 15 more minutes of yoga every day or start a meditation class.

463 **Nurturing breath** Deep, conscious breathing increases your intake of oxygen and prana, and expels toxins, refreshing your entire being. Expand your lungs as you inhale; when it feels as though they are at full capacity, gently add in one tenth more air, but do not force it. Then, when your lungs *feel* empty once you exhale, expel an extra tenth of stale air.

464 **Heart-centred affirmation** Hold **Lotus Mudra (273)**, a symbol of openness, then imagine the bud of a lotus flower in the centre of your chest. Inhaling, see the bud absorb light and blossom. To enhance your sense of self-nurturing, repeat the phrase, "I am open to transforming light." Exhale.

465 **Heart chakra mantra** The *bija mantra*, or seed sound, of the heart chakra, is *YAM* (pronounced "yum"). Quietly sing this mantra when you feel the need for some comfort from within.

466 **Happy in your own company** Make sure that you block out regular time in your calendar to spend alone. Yogis perceive that one of the paths to self-knowledge is solitude.

467   **A healthy ego** *Ahamkara* is the yogic term for the individual self. Yoga philosophy does not, as many people think, expect you to suppress this sense of self. Instead, you should nurture it: a solid ego means a strong sense of self-identity. Regard your ego for what it is – just one facet of your vast mind.

468   **Think positive** When you feel in any way vulnerable or in need of comfort, repeat a *sankalpa* – a short, positive phrase – that makes you feel as you would like to feel. Try, "I am worthy of others. They accept me as I am."

469   **Build supportive friendships** Aim to surround yourself with people who affirm you, and politely remove yourself from situations in which you feel uncomfortable or demeaned.

470   **THE RIGHT KIND OF NURTURING** *"Be careful what you water your dreams with. Water them with worry and fear and you will produce weeds that choke the life from your dream. Water them with optimism and solutions and you will cultivate success."*
LAO TZU (c.604–c.531BCE), CHINA

471 **Balanced living** In order to thrive, a plant needs the right amount of fresh air, natural light and warmth. So do you! Make sure your environments are *sattwic* – healthy. Start by opening windows, and avoiding harsh lighting and extreme temperatures.

472 **Nurture a flower** Buy a single flower and spend a few minutes a day contemplating it: let it remind you of the love, energy and care that you yourself require, and offer yourself this through yoga.

473 **Prepare your feet** Leave a little time before your next asana practice to nurture your feet by washing, exfoliating and moisturizing them with naturally fragranced products.

474 **Natural threads** Wear natural fabrics for asana practice, such as silk and organic cotton. These allow your skin to breathe.

475 **Listen to your body** When doing asanas, aim to tune into and respond to the messages your body sends: it might urge you to open up, push yourself harder or tell you that you're trying too hard. Remember that your body knows what's best for you.

476   **Nurturing practice** When you hold a yoga pose, visualize warm, comforting energy circulating through every part of you.

Foam blocks (477) To make certain seated poses feel more nurturing and achievable, invest in a few foam yoga blocks. Place them under your sitting bones to lift and release your hips.

478   **Nourish your upper body** If you crave emotional restoration, hold poses that drop your head below your heart, such as **Downward Dog Pose (481)** and **Shoulderstand (843)**, to bathe the upper body in freshly oxygenated blood and rest the heart.

479   **Faithful friends** Think of **Downward Dog Pose (481)** as an old friend who can offer you sage advice on your state of both body and mind. "Inhabit" it with focused awareness. What does it encourage your body to tell you today?

480   **Head-to-knee Pose** *Janu Sirsasana* To nourish your mind, sit on the floor, left leg straight and right leg bent, knee pointing out, heel to groin. Exhaling, fold over your left leg and reach to your feet for 2–3 minutes. Repeat on the other side, then relax. **>** 481

DOWNWARD DOG POSE

Adho Mukha Svanasana

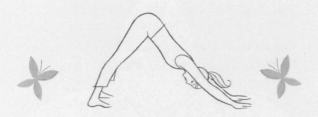

This posture, which is both a forward bend and a semi-inversion, requires you to look downward (*adho*) with your face (*mukha*) to resemble a dog stretching. It is an especially nurturing pose.

Come into a table-top shape as in **Cat Pose (45)**, tuck your toes under, and, as you inhale, dip your spine into a slightly concave backbend. Exhaling, push into your hands, lift your sitting bones and straighten your legs, to create an inverted "V". Draw your shoulder blades apart, lift your tail-bone and stretch your belly. After 10 breaths, rest in **Child's Pose (864).** 483

482 Benefit from sitting All seated poses have a meditative quality that standing poses do not. **Seated Twist (619)** and **Half Spinal Twist (817)** also care for your body from the inside out: they massage the internal organs, flush out toxins and bathe the viscera with fresh blood. Hold for several minutes.

483 Legs-up-the-wall Pose *Viparita Karani* To come into this restorative pose, place the long side of a bolster next to a wall and lie on the floor, facing the wall, with your legs extended up it. Bend your knees, and slide the bolster underneath your pelvis in order to elevate and support your hips. Relaxing your upper body, place your arms wide enough to permit easy breathing. If this is comfortable, hold the pose for several minutes and then relax. It will leave you feeling rested and revitalized. ❯ 506

484 Rest the senses In upward-facing restorative poses, such as **Legs-up-the-wall Pose (483)** or **Corpse Pose (931)**, put on an eye mask or wrap a scarf around your eyes to achieve *pratyahara*, withdrawal of the senses, yoga's fifth limb (see page 15).

DEVELOPING FLEXIBILITY

485   **TWO IN ONE** *"Flexible body, flexible mind."*
YOGIC PROVERB

486   **A flexible connection** Mental flexibility and inner spaciousness are the core work of yoga, equipping you to engage fully with others and to understand your place in the world. A flexible body is a joyous by-product of that process.

487   **Understanding postures** Watch carefully the journey that both your mind and your body take as you practise yoga asanas. Regular yoga sessions not only stretch and release your muscles but also quiet your mind, which prepares you both physically and mentally for the art of meditation – another extremely important part of yoga.

---

488   **A FAR-SEEING, FLEXIBLE MIND**
"One whose mind is stilled by the practice of yoga sees the self through the pure mind and rejoices in the self."
BHAGAVAD GITA (400–300BCE), INDIA

489 **Mind-body flexibility** The body and mind mirror each other: your way of moving reflects unconscious patterns of thought and behaviour, and vice versa. When you re-educate the body's connective tissue to slide in asanas rather than to adhere and tug, you boost your mental flexibility, too. This increased ability to go with the flow can be highly useful in relations with others.

490 **SUPPLE MIND** *"... oil your mind and your manners, to give them the necessary suppleness and flexibility; strength alone will not do ..."* LORD CHESTERFIELD (1694–1773), ENGLAND

491 **Avoiding stiffness** Beneath your skin lies an elastic but supportive "vest" of tissue, or "fascia", that protects your bones and muscles. Negative life experiences, such as physical injury and emotional trauma, as well as bad postural habits, can distort this vest, causing snags that restrict movement. As you undo these "snags" by regularly practising mindful asanas, the vest regains its ability to once more support, flex and release as it should, bringing about a sense not only a of physical freedom but also of emotional and mental flexibility.

492   **UNIVERSAL WISH** *"O, that this too too solid flesh would melt ..."*
WILLIAM SHAKESPEARE (1564–1616), *HAMLET*, ENGLAND

493   **Awareness practice** As you move into, hold and come out
of asanas, remember that each movement is only possible as
a result of the amazing muscles in your body contracting and
lengthening. Observe how pairs of muscles work in harmony.
The body's musculature is linked in chains. Your awareness of
these encourages them to communicate even better.

494   **COMPLETE FOCUS** *"Awareness must be like the rays of the sun:
extending everywhere, illuminating all."*
B.K.S. IYENGAR (BORN 1918), INDIA

495   **Starting a session** One aim of asanas is to restore a sense of
length and space to the spine so that the body's muscles and
organs have adequate room to relax and do their respective jobs
with ease. **Mountain Pose (57)** encourages this well by simply
and correctly ordering the spine's muscles and bones. It is best
to start every standing sequence with this posture.

496 **Muscle strength** To maintain a healthy, youthful spine – powerful enough to support the body yet flexible enough to yield to pressure without being injured – keep the body's anti-gravity muscles, the *erector spinae* that tramline the spine, strong with **Stretching the East Pose (640)** and **Boat Pose (704)**.

497 **Balancing flexibility with stability** Don't get carried away by flexibility in your asana practice. Grounding and structure are the foundations. Yogis who are super flexible can often suffer injury – for example, by hyper-extending joints or misaligning the body.

498 **POWERFUL YIELDING**
"A tree that cannot bend will crack in the wind. Thus by Nature's own decree, the soft and gentle are triumphant."
LAO TZU (c.604–c.531BCE), CHINA

499   **Yoga variety** Too much repetition of the same physical exercise can isolate and stress the muscles and joints rather than liberating them or allowing them to work in harmony. While it's important to find an approach to yoga that you find inspiring and that benefits you as much as possible, it's also key not to get too stuck in any one groove – variety is the spice of life (and of yoga!).

500   **Pure yoga body** If you practise asanas with care and dedication, your muscles and connective tissue will, with time, realign, unsnag and wrap around your joints in a balanced way – ensuring optimum muscle function. As your muscular structure becomes more balanced, any emotional imbalances, too, are likely to start settling naturally, which will allow you to invest more energy into relationships.

501   **A FLEXIBLE END-PLACE**

"One who is established in a comfortable posture while concentrating on the inner Self naturally becomes immersed in the Heart's ocean of bliss."
SIVA SUTRAS (EARLY 9TH CENTURY), INDIA

[203]

502 **Building flexibility** If you're new to yoga asanas and finding **Downward Dog Pose (481)** too challenging, then it may help to bend your knees in this pose, pressing your belly onto your thighs and rising onto your tip-toes to create a wave of energy that liberates your spine and frees your hamstrings. This is "Downward-facing Puppy" Pose.

503 **Willingness to yield** However experienced you are at yoga, there will be times when your muscles feel tight. Retain the mental flexibility, and humility, to adjust your poses according to your needs, such as by bending your knees in forward bends.

504 **Tuned shoulders** Yogis think of the arms as levers that, once lubricated with activity, free up energy in the heart region – the place from which we reach out to others. After sitting at a computer for hours, limber your shoulders (see p24), then practise **Eagle Pose (321)** and **Face of Light Pose (761)**.

505 **Free breathing** Tight clothing can hamper breathing as well as flexibility, so remember to wear loose items for asana practice.

BRIDGE POSE

Setu Bandha

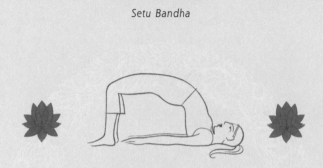

In this pose your body bends into the shape of a bridge (*setu* in Sanskrit), increasing spine flexibility and opening the front of the body, helping energy to flow to your heart chakra (see p18).

Lie on your back with your knees bent, and your feet hip-width apart and parallel. Breathe in deeply, lift your hips and chest upward, resting your body weight between your shoulders and your feet. Stretch your arms along the floor toward your heels. Think about lifting your heart and kidney area skyward. After several breaths, lower your back carefully, then relax. ➤ 534

507 **Softened gaze** When you're tense, notice how your eyes feel – probably hard and fixed? Yoga theory explains that because your external self reflects your internal self, "hard eyes" may relate to 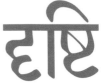 tension at the front of the brain. Consciously "soften" and widen your eyes and gaze, or *drishti* (see Sanskrit above), any time you feel stressed; sense your mind, too, "softening" as you do this.

508 **Widen your vision** Yoga teaches that relaxing the eyes helps you to cultivate an observing quality of mind: you'll be able to "see" around metaphorical corners and be more artful in communication. Both of these qualities are likely to increase your flexibility when you're dealing with other people.

509 **Soft eyes, soft diaphragm** As you relax and "soften" your eyes, your diaphragm, too, tends to "soften". This primary breathing muscle, beneath your lungs, stretches like a parachute as you inhale. When it's soft and flexible, you'll be able to breathe more freely and deeply – which boosts mental flexibility.

510 **Open-mind exercise** Hold one hand, palm up and place a coin on it. You don't need to grasp it; just observe how it sits there – in a "non-grasping" state known as *aparigraha*. Now make a fist and turn it downward, locking the coin within your fingers. Notice how tension arises and, if you open your hand to release the tension, the coin will fall. Aim to keep your mind as relaxed as an open palm, and you'll be able to receive gifts offered to you, whether a smile, an act of kindness or a job opportunity.

511 **Bridge visualization** Sit down, close your eyes and picture a bridge: visualize what it looks like, what lies beneath and above it, and what lies at either end of it: possibly lots of activity at one end and a calm, peaceful scene at the other. Walk slowly across it, observing any emotions that arise. This cultivates the flexibility of mind to take you from one quality of awareness to another – from gross to subtle – when dealing with other people.

512 **JUST A CROSSING POINT** *"Life is a bridge. Cross over it, but build no house on it."*
INDIAN PROVERB

PURITY AND HARMONY

513   **CLEAR VISION** *"Simply look with a pure heart. Not for reasons, nor explanations. In that way you will smash the ball of doubt."*
ZEN SAYING

514   **Cultivate purity** Practising asanas and pranayama regularly helps to break down old, unhelpful patterns – both physical and mental – allowing space for a clearer perception, unbiased by conditioned responses. Bring this pure, unburdened state of mind into your relations with others and you're likely to transform personal dynamics – whether with colleagues, friends or family.

515   **Lake meditation** Sit comfortably with your spine upright and close your eyes. Visualize your mind as a deep lake, and view passing thoughts as ripples on the surface of the water. Now dip beneath the surface, to the depths where the water is calm. Breathe in the peace and stillness of these depths. Then open your eyes, in the knowledge that this still place is always inside.

516   **Pure meditation** Only once you meditate every day will the mind really start to feel clearer: set aside 20 minutes each morning.

517 **Detached awareness** The yogic way of becoming more pure in your reactions to others is simple: always try to take a step back mentally from the dramas in your life. This keeps you still and focused, and stops you being washed away on waves of emotion.

---

518 **DROP ANCHOR**
"As a strong wind sweeps away a boat on the water, so the mind dwelling on even one of the senses carries away the intelligence."
BHAGAVAD GITA (400–300BCE), INDIA

---

519 **Pure compassion** Withdrawing from emotions (known as detachment in Buddhism) does not, paradoxically, mean hardening your heart. On the contrary, the practice of detachment, which includes not passing judgment on others or their actions, tends to create a purity of vision that draws the heart toward compassion.

520 **A CLEAR FOCUS** *"For the eye altering, alters all."*
WILLIAM BLAKE (1757–1827), ENGLAND

521 **Energy-cleansing** One aim of yoga is to purify the main energy channels (*nadis*), so that prana, or life energy, can freely ascend through the chakra system (see pp16–18), bringing about a harmonious state of being. **Alternate Nostril Breathing (69)** is one of the best ways to work toward this.

522 **Cloak visualization** Sit with your spine straight and eyes closed. Rest your hands on your thighs, palms up. Visualize a pillar of light-energy above you and feel it pouring down through the crown of your head. Imagine it filling your spine and filtering through all your cells. Then, imagine the rays expanding beyond your physical body to cocoon you in a cloak of light. Allow this cloak to protect you from the harshness of the external world and thus to maintain your own internal harmony.

523 **Your inner teacher** Yogis stress the importance of searching for your inner guru, or *satguru*, who allows you to see "the truth within" . Locate the hidden voice of this guru and listen and respond to what it says not only as you practise asanas and pranayama, but also as you go about your daily life.

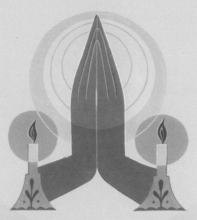

524 **Prayer Mudra** *Atmanjali Mudra* or *Namaste Mudra* Place your
palms together in the centre of your chest, fingers pointing
upward, and close your eyes. Offer this gesture to yourself, saying
the greeting "*Namaste*", meaning "I bow to you". By making this
symbol of peace and harmony, you give reverence to the *satguru*,
your inner guru, or the light within your heart. Offer it to others,
at yoga class and beyond, to celebrate the light in their hearts,
and so to cultivate compassion and harmonious relations.

525 **ME AND MY SHADOW** *"When the mind is pure, joy follows like a shadow that never leaves."*
THE BUDDHA (c.563–c.483BCE), INDIA

526 **An outside practice** When you feel in need of an increased sense of inner harmony, try practising yoga outside. Find a quiet spot – away from any superficial disturbances – so that not only the feeling of fresh air on your skin but also the awe-inspiring sights and sounds of pure nature can infuse your practice.

527 **Victorious Breath** *Ujjayi* As well as helping to deepen yoga practice, this breathing method is useful when you need to soothe your nerves – for example, before a job interview. Breathe both in and out through your nose, slightly contracting the glottis at the back of your throat so that you can hear your breath flowing. Do not force or tighten the throat, simply create a deep, slow breathing sound, as sibilant as the waves on the sea.

528 **Moving with your breath** The Astanga Vinyasa style of hatha yoga (see p21) recommends you use **Victorious Breath (527)**

while performing its *vinyasas*, breath-synchronized sequences
of movements. This is believed to "harmonize" your nerves and
purify your mind. The Sun Salutation sequence (see pp28-31)
is a good place to start applying the technique.

---

529 UNTROUBLED SEA

*"One who is undisturbed by the flow of desires
finds peace, as the ocean – though filled by
incessant rivers – remains still."*
BHAGAVAD GITA (400–300BCE), INDIA

---

530   **Breath meditation** The sound of **Victorious Breath (527)**
invites the mind inward, so makes a good focus for meditation.
Sit with your spine upright and close your eyes. Begin *Ujjayi*
breathing, following your breath until it stills other thoughts and
makes your mind feel as spacious and pure as the sea. After a few
minutes, return to normal breathing and open your eyes. Try to
retain an awareness of this calm, internal ocean as you go about
your business today, returning there when the words or actions
of others make you feel agitated or disturbed.

531 **A practice that suits you** Like everything else, yoga will only enhance your life if you approach it in a way that suits your own mind and body. If you're stressed, for example, you may be best advised to avoid a vigorous physical practice that fires you up, and opt instead for a few deep stretches, such as **Cat Pose (45)** and **Seated Twist (619),** followed by the "yogic sleep" **Yoga Nidra (940)**. Listen to what **Your inner teacher (523)** advises.

---

532 **SEE UNITY IN THE MANY**
"Approach life with a mind sharpened by your practices, and see the One in the many."
UPANISHADS (800–400BCE), INDIA

---

533 **Tailormade yoga** You might like to try the Viniyoga method of yoga – which evolved out of the teachings of T. Krishnamacharya and T.K.V. Desikachar. This school focuses on carefully tailoring *vinyasas* (sequences of poses and breathing) to meet individual needs. Its intuitive teachers may help to guide you toward a highly personal practice that can transform your relationship with both yourself and others.

TRIANGLE POSE
Trikonasana

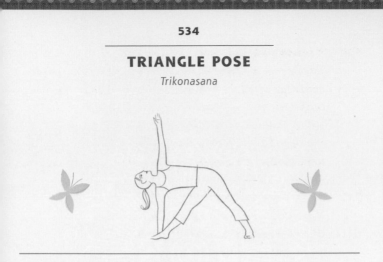

This pose bends your body to resemble a triangle (*trikona* in Sanskrit), opening up your entire front side and thus encouraging a harmonious flow of prana.

Stand with your feet 1m (3ft) wide and outstretch your arms. Turn your left foot in, internally rotating the thigh. Turn your right foot out 90 degrees, externally rotating the thigh. Exhaling, stretch to your right and place your right hand on the floor beside your little toe (or on a yoga block). Stretch your left arm up. Take a few breaths. Come up, switch sides, then relax. ➤ 549

535 **Sea-bed visualization** Sit upright or lie in **Corpse Pose (931)**, close your eyes and imagine diving down through a deep ocean. At the bottom is a layer of debris – your store of memories. Sift through it. Don't be disturbed by any ugly creatures that lurk there. Direct your gaze instead to the glimmering fragments of minerals and gold – your precious thoughts. Brush off the sludge and set this pure treasure free from the debris, allowing it to bubble up into the water and drift to the surface. Let these precious thoughts illuminate your relations with others.

536   **Words from the heart** Yogis advise us to "listen with the
throat", meaning to be receptive and only speak when it is likely
to be useful – an acquired practice that is rare in our culture of
incessant chatter. When interacting with others, try always to
speak from a pure heart, with words that promote harmony.

537   **Throat meditation** Lie comfortably in **Corpse Pose (931)**,
close your eyes and take your awareness to your throat, which in
yogic thought symbolizes purity and heartfelt communication.
Consciously relax your throat: imagine it dropping to the back of
your neck, open, unrestricted and spacious. Visualize turquoise
light (the colour of the throat chakra) bathing it, bringing the
healing you need to connect on a deeper level with others.

538   **Paths to harmony** To embody the eight-limbed yogic path
considered to lead to inner harmony, it is important to give the
mind just as much attention as the body when practising yoga
asanas. It can be useful to get into the habit of ending every
asana session with a visualization to encourage the mind to settle,
such as **Light yourself up (238)** or **Mind-cave focus (298)**.

539 **Yogis and yoginis** Modern yoga is neither a path for men only nor women only, as male and female energies are revered for their complementary qualities. *Yogi* is the name given to a male practitioner of yoga; *yogini* is his female equivalent.

540 **Female energy** In yoga theory, *shakti* is the name given to creative life-energy, which is feminine. It forms one of the poles of energy that governs the universe. Shakti is also another name for Hindu goddess of life Devi, consort of the god Shiva.

541 **Male energy** *Shiva* is the name given to the masculine energy that channels the female creative life-force in the universe. You might like to think of it as the container for the female life essence. Shiva is also an important Hindu creator god.

542 **The divine feminine** The tantric yoga tradition primarily worships the female creative spirit, Shakti – feminine energy being considered higher in spiritual awareness than masculine energy. All of us, however, have feminine, Shakti energy within us, irrespective of our gender.

543 SHIVA'S TRIBUTE TO SHAKTI
"With thee I can create all things
Without thee I am powerless."
S'MRIMAD DEVI BHAGAWATAM (AFTER 200BCE)

---

544   Nadi visualization Hatha yoga considers that the two poles of
energy in the universe – feminine and masculine – are reflected in
the body by two main energy channels, the *ida* (lunar) and *pingala*
(solar) *nadis* that weave around the spine. To gain an understanding
of these qualities, rest your gaze on an image of the two channels
(369), thinking about logic at the masculine, solar channel,
and intuition at the feminine, lunar channel. Consider how they
complement and support one another in your life.

545   Shiva Mudra In this whole-body mudra, you adopt the qualities
of the god Shiva standing in a stable, open-hearted way. Standing,
slightly bend your right leg, lift your left foot and hook it behind
your right calf. Raise your right hand to shoulder level in front,
palm facing out. Point your left hand down by your left hip, palm
facing backward. Hold for 10 breaths, switch sides, then relax.

546 **Goddess of Life Mudra** *Shakti Mudra*
When your intuitive energy reserves,
or *shakti*, need boosting,
tuck your thumbs into their
respective palms and drape
your index and middle
fingers over them. Straighten
your ring and little fingers and
bring your hands together
so that your fingertips and
knuckles meet. Hold for
several breaths and release
with a long exhalation,
or *langhana*.

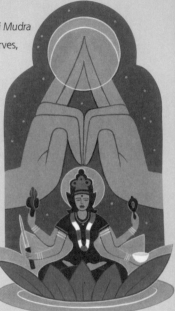

547 **Words of intuition** To
further enhance intuitive
energy within, say the following
words as you hold **Goddess of Life Mudra
(546)**: "Harmony and silence fill my being".

548   **Sacral chakra meditation** Sit quietly, close your eyes and focus on your pelvis, the site of the second, or *swadhisthana*, chakra (see p17). Breathe deeply into this energy centre, which governs sexuality and creativity. Giving it this attention will enhance your capacity for loving expression and bonding with others.

549   **Butterfly Pose** *Baddha Konasana* This pose energizes the sensual chakra, *swadhisthana*, in your pelvis area. Sit on the floor, with the soles of your feet together, knees out to the side, holding your toes with your hands. Move your knees up and down like wings, keeping your spine straight. Then relax ➤ 591

550   **Body poetry** Evocative use of language doesn't only inspire the mind and enrich the senses but also inspires the body, so think up poetic ways to describe your movements as you do asanas.

     Language exploration (551) Consider the following example of playful, evocative language to help to give you a sense of groundedness when you next practise a seated posture: "Your sitting bones are pomegranates, the stolen fruit of the underworld. Let them return from whence they came!"

552   **Spine visualization** The spine carries messages to and from your brain to the many muscles in your body and houses your energy centres, or chakras. "Awakening" the spine through physical movement (in the form of asanas) therefore encourages prana to flow more smoothly throughout the body, opening the chakras. During asanas, visualize the spine as an estuary that leads to a hidden ocean of energy within, referred to by some yogis as "the pulse of the morning rivers".

553   **HEIGHTENING THE SENSES**
"Oh! That you could turn your eyes toward the napes of your necks, and make but an interior survey of your good selves."
WILLIAM SHAKESPEARE (1564–1616), *CORIOLANUS*, ENGLAND

554   **Nourish sight** In order to function fully as you interact in daily life, the delicate muscles of your eyes require rest now and again from constant external onslaught. When they ache and you feel frazzled by contact with the outside world, recline for 20 minutes wearing an eye mask, and repeat the mantra *soham* **(7)** to soothe your other senses.

555   **Tibetan-bell meditation** *Nada yoga* is the yoga of sound. Sit
in a quiet place, where interruptions are unlikely, and chime an
old-fashioned bell. Let the sound waves reverberate inside you
– imagine the sound cleansing your sense organs.

556   **Recognize the love in your life** Take regular time out from
all the goings-on around you to reflect, re-gather yourself and
contemplate those who offer you love and support in your life.

557   **What is love?** The spiritual teacher Osho points out that the
desire to seek love from others tends to stem from an emptiness
in our own heart. Rather than asking yourself questions about
your relationships with others, delve deeper into your relationship
with yourself – this is *jnana yoga*, self-enquiry (see p13).

---

558   **LOVE IS A LONGING FOR THE INFINITE**
*"Verily, not for the sake of the husband himself
is a husband dear, but for the love of the Soul
in the husband that a husband is dear."*
BRIHAD-ARANYAKA UPANISHAD (800–400BCE), INDIA

LIVING IN HARMONY

559   OUR ONE WORLD *"The whole universe is your home.*
All are your family."
SRI NEEM KAROLI BABA (DIED 1973), INDIA

560   Yoga, the great leveller Yoga is for everyone, regardless of
occupation, social status or age. Whether you're a business tycoon,
a baker or a bus driver, it's a joy to be part of a yoga class where
everyone practises together, without worldly labels.

561   A yoga community While personal practice is essential for
developing strong, flexible asanas, practising in a community of
others is a grounding experience that helps you to explore other
yoga paths, such as *karma* yoga, selfless service (see p13).

562   Bonds of love *"When everybody in the world loves one another,*
then the weak will not be overpowered by the strong, the few will
not be oppressed by the many, the poor will not be mocked by the
wealthy, the humble will not be disdained by the honoured, and
the simple will not be deceived by the cunning."
MOTSI (c.470–c.390BCE), CHINA

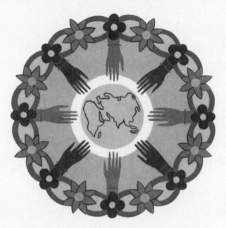

563 **Welcoming classes** Look for classes that offer the warmth and
compassion of a yoga *shala*, Sanskrit for a sanctuary or refuge.

564 **INVOCATION FOR YOGA CLASS**
*"Let us attain vitality together. Let our study be
inspiring. Let there be harmony between us.
OM, peace, peace, peace."*
KAIVALYA UPANISHAD (800–400BCE), INDIA

565 **Yoga for everyone** Yoga is not only for the young, fit or supple. Encourage your grandparents to do some gentle exercises, such as **Mountain Pose (57)** and **Palm Tree Pose (117)**, or to simply sit on a chair and bend forward or lift their arms overhead.

566 **A subtle thread** Notice how, as yoga helps you to integrate your mind, body and spirit, it also takes you on an outward journey toward a sense of connection with all beings.

567 **THE WEB OF LIFE** *"We cannot live only for ourselves. A thousand fibres connect us with our fellow men; and among those fibres, as sympathetic threads, our actions run as causes, and they come back to us as effects."*
HERMAN MELVILLE (1819–1891), USA

568 **Yoga trust exercise** Sit on the floor back to back with a partner. Press your backs against each other and bend your knees, tucking your heels close to your buttocks. Rest your arms by your sides, then firmly press your backs together, grounding your feet. Straighten your legs and rise up simultaneously.

569 **Yoga balance exercise** Stand back to back with a partner. Ask her to stay standing while you bend your knees, so that your buttocks are lower than hers. Interlink arms. Ask your partner to relax and to trust you, then carefully bend forward until your partner is lifted and balanced on your back in a passive backbend, possibly with her feet lifting slightly off the floor. Hold for several breaths. Carefully return to standing and change roles. (Avoid if either of you has a back problem or feels nervous.)

570 **Sense of connectedness** When you feel in need of comfort and harmony, gather together with friends and sit in a circle. Place your right palms up and left palms down, meeting palms with the next person to make a connecting thread that runs around the circle. Close your eyes and practise **Metta Meditation (457)** to promote loving-kindness.

571 **Time to move on** Good yoga teachers guide students to the best of their knowledge. Then, once they are ready, the teacher sets students free to continue their journey. Listen to your teacher if she suggests that you move on to pursue your study elsewhere.

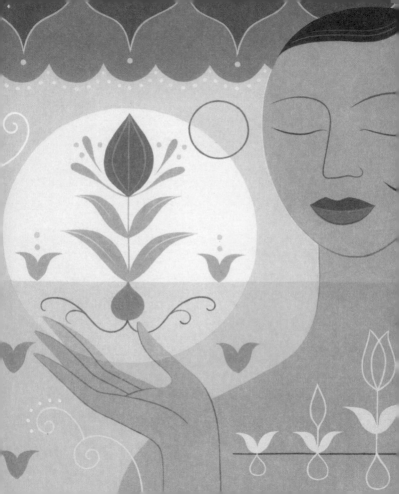

IN TIMES OF TROUBLE

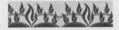

ACCEPTING CHANGE

572   **LIFE IS CHANGE** *"The way that we see things today does not have to be the way we saw them yesterday. That is because the situations, our relationships to them, and we ourselves have changed in the interim. This notion of constant change suggests that we do not have to be discouraged."*
T.K.V. DESIKACHAR (BORN 1938), INDIA

573   **Avoid grasping** Patanjali advises us in his Yoga Sutras to accept change. You can do this by adopting an approach of *aparigraha*, one of yoga's five *yamas*, or ethics (see p14). Meaning "non-grasping", this can be interpreted as not being possessive about things or people and therefore not trying to stop them changing.

574   **LET GO** *"When I let go of what I am, I become what I might be."*
LAO TZU (c.604–c.531BCE), CHINA

575   **Visualizing red** The colour red has an empowering effect when you meditate on it. Related to the element fire, it builds the confidence, courage and open-hearted warmth necessary to accept that people and situations change. Visualizing red also supports your heart, where release from any sense of "grasping" in life begins. Sit and close your eyes, concentrate on the *citta kash* (mind-screen) in front of your closed eyes and visualize a rich shade of red. Feel it empowering you to let go of assumptions.

576 **Relax your grip** Don't try to force changes in your body through asana practice: your body will resist. Instead, accept your body as it is, and change will follow in time, with a daily practice. Yoga philosophy says the same is true of relationships. Don't actively strive for change: let changes develop at their own pace.

577 **JUST OBSERVE THE WORLD** *"Sitting quietly, doing nothing, spring comes, and the grass grows by itself."*
ZEN SAYING

578 **Breathe free** When change is coming too fast – whether at work or at home – don't neglect your asana practice. Stretching helps you to breathe more deeply, which counters stress and encourages prana to flow more freely around your body, allowing you to thrive in the midst of change.

[231]

579 **Feel your sacral chakra**
Water is the element
associated with the
swadhisthana chakra (see
p17). Gazing at its *yantra*,
or visual representation (see
right), helps you to take on the
qualities of water, which flows on
no matter what obstacles it meets. Look
at its blue background, then close your eyes and imagine the
same watery fluidity in your own body's cells. When faced with
difficult changes, meditate on this yantra for a few moments.

580 **SPEND TIME HERE AND NOW** *"Do not dwell in the past, do not
dream of the future, concentrate the mind on the present moment."*
THE BUDDHA (c.563–c.483BCE), INDIA

581 **Value shades of grey** The Vedic texts (see p10) advocate
freedom from extremes, whether good or bad. You can work
toward this by trying not to judge or label people or events.

Stepping back and simply observing the world without passing judgment makes it easier to tolerate change and allows you to let go of old ways of thinking and to accept new ones.

---

582 LET GO OF RESULTS
"Act with a spirit of detachment, being equal to success or failure. Such evenness of mind is called yoga."
BHAGAVAD GITA (400–300BCE), INDIA

---

583 New growth visualization When change hurts, use this exercise to remind yourself that only through change are we able to evolve. Kneel in **Child's Pose (864)** and visualize yourself as a seed deep underground. Imagine the effort of pushing up through the hard ground, followed by the delight of emerging as a bud into the brightness and warmth of a new day.

584 BE BENDY *"Notice that the stiffest tree is the most easily cracked, while the bamboo or willow survives by bending with the wind."*
JAPANESE SAYING

585 **Ganesh contemplation** Ganesh is the Hindu elephant deity associated with overcoming physical and mental obstacles. Contemplate his picture, noticing how his physical characteristics reflect his ability to endure change. His large ears and small mouth show he listens rather than talks. His small eyes suggest he looks inward rather than out. His large stomach is able to digest everything, good or bad, while his axe severs the bonds preventing us from changing. Consider these qualities when you have obstacles to overcome.

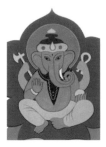

586 **Recognize your true nature** Ayurveda, the ancient Indian system of healing, teaches that each of us is born with a certain set of physical and emotional qualities, made up of the motivating principles, or *dosha*, constituting earth (*kapha*), fire (*pitta*) and air (*vata*). This elemental nature, or *prakriti*, shapes the way you react to challenges. A healthy individual has a combination of all three *dosha*, and practising certain asanas helps to balance them, equipping you to adapt better to change **(587–589)**.

587   **Earthy constitution and change** If your dominant *dosha* is earth (*kapha*), you tend to be slow-moving and calm. Although you're not easily riled by change, practising energizing, opening poses such as **Camel Pose (447)** and **Half Spinal Twist (817)** will help you to deal with any challenges that *do* come along.

588   **Fiery constitution and change** If your dominant *dosha* is fire (*pitta*), you tend to be strong, well-built and able to rise to change by thinking quickly, but you can be hot-headed. To cope better, reduce your stress with cooling poses such as **Head-to-knee Pose (480)** and **Wide-legged Seated Forward Bend (789)**.

589   **Airy constitution and change** If your dominant *dosha* is air (*vata*), you tend to be tall, lithe and easily irritated or worried by change. Ground yourself to cope better with **Alternate Nostril Breathing (69)** or **Krama breathing (185)**.

590   **Sit in stillness** Sit in **Hero Pose (591)** for a few minutes when you crave some stillness during tempestuous change. Physical steadiness helps to bring mental stability.

591 **Hero Pose** *Virasana* This pose exemplifies a heroic determination, stillness and focus that can help you to endure a whirlwind of change. From kneeling, sit on your buttocks between your feet; if your knees hurt, place a yoga block beneath your sitting bones. Point the soles of your feet up and spread the tops of your toes into the floor. Aim to draw your knees together, kneecaps facing forward. Rest your hands on your thighs, palms down, lengthen your spine and ground your sitting bones. Then relax. ❯ 592

592 **Hero Pose variation** To combat tension during times of unsettling change and create a sense of inner spaciousness, sit in **Hero Pose (591)** and extend your arms overhead, feeling a sense of length through the sides of your waist. Interlink your fingers and press your palms skyward. Feel the muscles between your ribs, the sides of your waist and your diaphragm stretch. Then relax. ❯ 619

593 **PRESENT IN CHANGE** *"Change, both good and bad, is inevitable, so try not to waste your energy either fighting or fearing it. Instead, aim to accept it as part of the natural cycle of birth, life and death."* GRAHAM STONES (BORN 1974), ENGLAND

594   **Gods of change** Three prominent Hindu gods symbolize a cycle of change in the natural world: Brahma, god of new life, stands for creation; Vishnu, preserver of life, symbolizes maintenance and balance; while Shiva, god of destruction, represents decay and regeneration. Look for these forces of change in action in the world around you – in the cycle of the seasons, for example, and also in our own life cycle. Seeing change in this way may help you to accept that every alteration in circumstance, however sad or traumatic at the time, is part of a natural cycle.

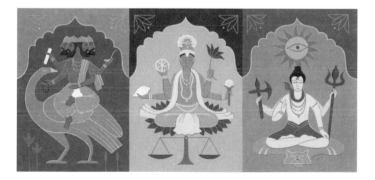

595 **An ever-changing body** Part of the joy of a regular asana practice is watching your body's alignment and energy levels change over time. As your physical alignment improves, you learn that your body is not a fixed entity, and is constantly evolving.

596 **EVER MOVING**
"Man's yesterday may ne'er be like his morrow;
Nought may endure but Mutability."
PERCY BYSSHE SHELLEY (1792–1822), ENGLAND/ITALY

597 **Women and change** Vary your yoga practice to reflect changes in your body during the month. On the first two days of menstruation, women should avoid strong, standing asanas and instead practise gentle hip-opening forward bends such as **Head-to-Knee Pose (480)** and **Butterfly Pose (549)**.

598 **Men and change** Yogis believe that men's energy cycles are linked to the sun's. Observe how your energy levels change throughout the year and adapt your practice to include restorative poses like **Legs-up-the-wall Pose (483)** when your energy wanes.

RESOLVING CONFLICT

599   **THE WISDOM OF FORESIGHT** *"Take control of events while they are peaceful. Prevent difficulties before they arise. Prepare for rough spots while the going is still smooth. Deal with the situation before it descends into chaos."*
LAO TZU (c.604–c.531BCE), CHINA

600   **Take time out** Before any brewing conflict that you can sense reaches a head, try to mentally step outside of the situation, into the spacious state of mind that is the aim of yoga – *buddhi*. You can do this by practising any asana, breathing or meditation technique in this book. Once you have opened the door to the *buddhi* state of mind, tensions will start to fall away.

601   **Nerve-soothing mantra** When something angers you, repeat the *bija mantra*, or seed sound, *SOM*. This is valued for soothing the nerves and encouraging a measured response.

602   **LET IT GO** *"Holding on to anger is like grasping a hot coal with the intent of throwing it at someone: you are the one who gets burned."*
THE BUDDHA (c.563–c.483BCE), INDIA

603 **Cleansing twisting poses** Twists wring out and re-energize the spine. As you practise **Twisting Triangle Pose (357)** or **Seated Twist (619)**, imagine squeezing out your tension. Each time you exhale, let go of anger and negativity. Each time you inhale, picture clear energy being absorbed into the left and right sides of your body – rebalancing them, for greater equanimity.

604 **LET TROUBLES GO** *"Let the past drift away with the water."*
JAPANESE SAYING

605   **Japa mantra** Ancient yogis taught that if you repeat a *bija mantra*, or seed sound, over and over (a process called *japa*), the sound resonates internally, bringing about subtle changes in consciousness. The mantra *GAM* (pronounced "gum") is invoked for dissolving mental blockages. Repeat it, breathing steadily and calmly, when your mind feels immobilized by conflict.

606   **ROAD MAP TO PEACE** *"Sow a thought and reap an action, sow an action and reap a habit, sow a habit and reap a character, sow a character and reap a destiny."*
SWAMI SIVANANDA (1887–1963), INDIA

607   **How did we get here?** The introspection involved in yoga practice can help you to retrace the path of decisions that brought you to a place of conflict. Knowing how you arrived at this place will hopefully show you the route back to solve the conflict.

608   **TAKE BACK YOUR WORDS** *"Humility is not cowardice. Meekness is not weakness. Humility and meekness are indeed spiritual powers."*
SWAMI SIVANANDA (1887–1963), INDIA

609   **Make peace** Isaiah 11.6 says that, *"The wolf ... shall dwell with the lamb"*. Visualize this when you need to make peace with "demons", either external or internal.

610   **INNER AND OUTER ENEMIES** *"When there is no enemy within, the enemies outside cannot hurt you."*
AFRICAN PROVERB

611   **The peace mudra** *Shambhavi Mudra* This is a symbolic gesture of peace made with the eyes. Yogis believe that it reduces stress and soothes the mind by restoring balance between the right and left sides of the brain. Sit comfortably with your spine straight, with your hands in *Jnana Mudra* **(96)**. Then draw your gaze in and up toward the centre of your forehead. Hold for several moments while observing your breathing, allowing this focus to calm your thoughts. Then relax. Stop if your eyes feel tense.

612   **Mantra for peace** To build inner peace at times of discord, whether due to friction at work or in your relationships, repeat the *bija mantra*, or seed sound, *SHAM* (pronounced "shum") daily.

613   **TURN THE OTHER CHEEK** *"Forget like a child any injury done by somebody immediately. Never keep it in the heart. It kindles hatred."* SWAMI SIVANANDA (1887–1963), INDIA

614   **Sweet talking** The master teacher of Astanga Vinyasa yoga, Sri K. Pattanda Jois, advises us not to be ruthless when telling harsh truths. All forms of yoga help you to develop tactful ways of communicating unpleasant matters truthfully, without cruelty.

615   **ACTING WITH KINDNESS**
"Be compassionate. Not just to your friends, but to everyone."
BHAGAVAD GITA (400–300BCE), INDIA

616   **Cooling practice** When you feel hot and bothered, opt for cooling asanas rather than overheating the body with *rajasic* (stimulating) activity. Hold poses for longer than usual and emphasize hip-openers such as **Butterfly Pose (549)**, forward bends such as **Stretching the West Pose (683)** and inverted poses such as **Downward Dog Pose (481)**.

617   **YOGA ON AND OFF THE MAT** *"There is a strong relationship between yoga on the mat and yoga off the mat. I've come to recognize that the energy generated in practice allows me to find clarity amid the conflicting thoughts in my mind."*
GRAHAM STONES (BORN 1974), ENGLAND

618   **Cosmic head-butt** The Hindu gods of creation (Brahma), maintenance (Vishnu) and destruction (Shiva) epitomize the three *gunas*, or qualities, that yogis perceive to be latent in all matter: the force of creation (*rajas*), balance (*sattwa*) and decline (*tamas*). If you feel confused about a course of action, you may feel these energies are in opposition within you, as if the gods were engaged in a cosmic head-butt! Try to regard this not as extremes causing internal unrest, but as polarities that offer creative potential for the resolution of internal conflict. You can then work toward balancing *tamas* and *rajas* in your asana practice, and beyond, in order to achieve the balance of *sattwa*.

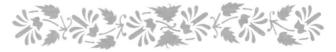

SEATED TWIST POSE

Bharadvajasana

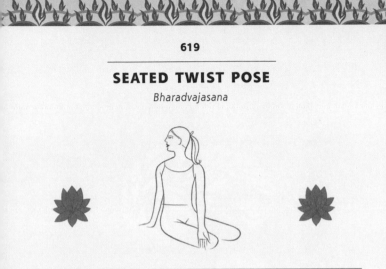

Bharadvaja was one of the seven legendary *rishi* (sages) said to have composed the hymns of the Vedas (see pp10–11). Doing this pose calls on his great wisdom to help you to reconcile any conflict in your life.

Kneel on the floor, with your buttocks resting on your heels, and then drop your hips to the right of your feet. Twisting to the right, place your left hand on your right knee. Twist to the right, placing your right hand on the floor pointing backward, behind your right hip. Hold this position, breathing evenly. Release, repeat to the left, then relax. ▶ 640

LIFTING THE BLUES

620   YOU HAVE THE POWER TO FLY

"Be like the bird who, halting in her flight,
On boughs too slight,
Feels them give way beneath her,
Yet sings, knowing she hath wings."
VICTOR HUGO (1802–1885), FRANCE

621   Come home to yoga When you're feeling low for any reason,
a regular yoga session at a set time of day and for a set length
of time is more valuable and supportive than ever, as it provides
you with a much-needed positive focus.

622   Surrender to the divine Forward-bending poses, such as
Head-to-Knee Pose (480), induce a form of introspection
that can be nurturing when the blues strike. Consciously
surrender yourself to the care of a higher power while in the
pose. Letting go to this force, *ishwara pranidhana*, is the final
niyama of the second limb of the eight-fold path (see p14)
and the highest attitude we aim for in yoga. As you do this,
repeat to yourself: "I relax into happiness."

623   FINDING TRUST IN THE PATH *"If a man wishes to be sure of the path he treads on, he must close his eyes and walk in the dark."* ST JOHN OF THE CROSS (1542–1591), SPAIN

624   Finding the light During "dark" periods, your asana and meditation practice offer you not only safe, quiet time out but also the opportunity to explore your thoughts and process your emotions. Yogis believe that taking time out in this way allows you to emerge into the light as a more complete person.

625   Curl up When you feel low and vulnerable, explore nurturing **Child's Pose (864)**. As you kneel, fold your spine over your thighs and curl up like a fern, turning your mind inward, away from your worries. Simply rest here, feeling the security and protection that the pose brings. Imagine all negativity sweeping away over your back. Emerge when your mind feels clearer.

626   BEACON IN THE DARK *"Truly, it is in darkness that one finds the light, so when we are in sorrow, then this light is nearest to all of us."* MEISTER ECKHART (1260–1328), GERMANY

627 **Torches of wisdom** *Swadhaya*, spiritual study, is an important part of the eight-limbed yoga path (see p14). To temper sadness, learn more about a prophet, saint or guru who appeals to you, such as Krishna, Jesus or Mohammed. Draw inspiration from them and feel a little of their light illuminate you and your actions. Let this light shine into the world.

628 **ASK FOR ILLUMINATION**
"Be thou unto me a light, O Krishna, in my darkness. I ask thee to dispel this doubt in me."
BHAGAVAD GITA (400–300BCE), INDIA

629 **Nature's cure** Increased exposure to natural light helps to lift the blues in some people, so try practising yoga outside.

   Explore the nightscape (630) When you're unable to sleep, let the glow of the stars and moon calm your troubled mind.

631 **CONTRASTS** *"When it is dark enough, you can see the stars."*
RALPH WALDO EMERSON (1803–1882), USA

632   THE EVERLASTING SEASON

"Spring has its hundred flowers, Autumn its moon.
Summer has its cooling breezes, Winter its snow.
If you allow no idle concerns
To weight on your heart,
Your whole life will be one
Perennial good season."

ZEN POEM

633   Lotus contemplation Tantric philosophy teaches that
contemplating a lotus at difficult times brings
spiritual growth. Imagine the radiant beauty
of a lotus whose stem extends from a swamp.
Consider how the flower draws nourishment
from the murky depths yet remains pristine.
How can you make this true in your life?

634   Buy flowers Tantra teaches that indulging in pleasures helps us
to avoid thoughts of past woes and future anxieties, and to live in
the present. Buy yourself flowers to connect to the beauty of now.

635   **Value play** When you feel dragged down by worries at the end of a working day, be gentle with yourself. This is *ahimsa* (non-violence), which can be as simple as doing something you love instead of obsessing over things you view as having gone wrong.

636   **Natural lift** *"Our minds need relaxation and give way,*
Unless we mix with work a little play."
MOLIÈRE (1622–1673), FRANCE

637   **What makes you sad?** When we rely on the accumulation of material goods to bring about happiness, it can breed an insatiable desire for more, making us feel sad and leaving a spiritual void. Fill this void with spiritual pursuits such as yoga.

   Happy place (638) Remember that all yoga leads you to regard happiness as an inner quality, not an external commodity.

639   **COMPOSITION OF HAPPINESS** *"The happiness of life ...*
is made up of minute fractions – the little, soon-forgotten charities
of a kiss, a smile, a kind look, a heartfelt compliment."
SAMUEL TAYLOR COLERIDGE (1772–1834), ENGLAND

STRETCHING THE EAST POSE

Purvottanasana

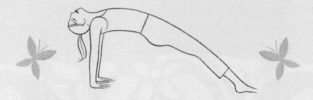

This pose opens the front of the body, its "east side" in yoga.
It also encourages emotional lightness when you feel weighed down,
and strengthens your ability to bear a heavy load.

Sit on the floor with your legs stretched forward and your spine straight. Place your hands on the floor behind you, fingers facing forward. Inhaling, lift your body into a diagonal "plank" shape. Press the soles of your feet down into the ground and your big toes together. Take 5–10 deep breaths. Release and curl into **Child's Pose (864)** to counterstretch, then relax. ❯ 674

641 **Beating the blues** When you feel emotionally detached and lethargic, cultivate "inner fire" with a warming practice of Sun Salutations (see pp28–31), twists such as **Twisting Triangle (357)** and backbends such as **Camel Pose (447)**.

642 **Visualization for SAD**
To combat Seasonal Affective Disorder, close your eyes and visualize a bright light, or *jyoti* (see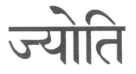

Sanskrit, right), perhaps orange or yellow. Let this flood onto the *citta kash* (mind-screen) in front of your closed eyes, then wash through your body, brightening any areas that feel "closed in".

643 **UNCLOUD YOUR VISION** *"Some day perhaps the inner light will shine forth from us, and then we'll need no other light."*
JOHN WOLFGANG VON GOETHE (1749–1832), GERMANY

644 **Sun salute** The Sun Salutation's traditional 12 steps (see p29) attune you to the stimulating power of the sun. Practise them as a sequence to start the day in a positive frame of mind.

645   **LEARN TO COPE** *"Better to light a candle than curse the darkness."*
CHINESE PROVERB

646   **Solar tuning** To tune into mood-enhancing solar energy when
doing the traditional Sun Salutation sequence, accompany each
of the 12 key movements with the **Sun Salutation Mantras
(647)** used by the Sivananda and Satyananda schools of yoga.

647   **Sun Salutation Mantras** **1** *Salutations to the friend of all.*
2 *Salutations to the shining one.* **3** *Salutations to the source of
creation.* **4** *Salutations to the One who illuminates.* **5** *Salutations to
the One who moves through the sky.* **6** *Salutations to the giver of
strength and nourishment.* **7** *Salutations to the golden cosmic womb.*
8 *Salutations to the rays of the sun.* **9** *Salutations to the infinite cosmic
mother.* **10** *Salutations to the rising sun.* **11** *Salutations to the source
of life energy.* **12** *Salutations to the one who leads to enlightenment.*

648   **End mantra** To seal in the positive effects of the Sun Salutation
sequence, end with the Sanskrit mantra *"OM, shanti, shanti, shanti"*,
which translates as *"OM, peace, peace, peace".*

RELIEVING ANXIETY

649 **LOOK WITHIN** *"Peace comes from within. Do not seek it without."*
THE BUDDHA (c.563–c.483BCE), INDIA

650 **Turn to Patanjali** Read the opening aphorisms of Patanjali's
Yoga Sutras to find out how yoga helps to focus the mind and
soothe anxiety. Sutra 2 affirms that: *"Yoga is the stilling of the
thought waves of the mind."*

651 **Identify obstacles to contentment** Patanjali describes in the
Yoga Sutras the *klesas*, or obstacles, that shatter a cool, calm state
of mind: *"... illness, dullness, doubt, negligence, laziness, not desisting
from self-destructive habits, mistaken perception, not being grounded,
and instability."* Consider which of these apply to you, if any.
What could you do to counter them?

652 **Modern foes** Financial pressures gnaw at many of us, boosting
stress levels. The yoga way is to live moderately, within your
means, and not to enter into debt. Cut up paid-off store cards,
avoid credit arrangements and pay with cash whenever possible,
keeping receipts to monitor your spending habits.

653   **SIMPLIFY FOR PEACE OF MIND** *"Every increased possession loads us with a new weariness."*
JOHN RUSKIN (1819–1900), ENGLAND

654   **Value the real** A materialistic lifestyle can create anxiety by constantly causing you to covet new goods. Yoga urges you to focus instead on your spiritual life, which is everlasting.

655   **FIND PERMANENCE** *"Knowing all objects to be impermanent, let not their contact blind you, resolve again and again to be aware of the Self that is permanent."*
SRI TIRUMALAI KRISHNAMACHARYA (1888–1989), INDIA

656   **Anxiety-relieving mudra** *Bhuchari Mudra* This gesture, made with the eyes, eases anxiety and protects your memory from the effects of stress. Sit upright facing a white wall. Place your right thumb between your nose and top lip. Point your little finger up between your eyes and stare at its tip. After a moment, move your finger from here, gaze into the space where it was and let the concentration clear your mind.

657   **Ponder big questions** If your anxiety stems from an onslaught of tiny worries, put them in perspective by asking yourself big questions. What is the purpose of life? Why are we here? Reading the yoga texts (see p11) may help you to address these questions.

658   **LET THE SMALL STUFF GO** *"... do not be anxious about your life, what you shall eat or what you shall drink, nor about your body, what you shall put on. Is not life more than food, and the body more than clothing? Look at the birds of the air: they neither sow nor reap nor gather into barns, and yet your heavenly Father feeds them."*
THE GOSPEL OF ST MATTHEW 6.25–26

659   **Nourish your mind** Sivananda yoga says that to beat anxiety we must nourish the mind with "right thinking", one of yoga's five pillars (see p23). One way of doing this is by meditating on a mandala – a symbolic picture or pattern, such as the Buddha image opposite, that represents the cosmos. The circular shape of a mandala can also be understood as a symbol of wholeness, unity and the infinite. Use it to help you to find your calm, centred self when life's worries get too much.

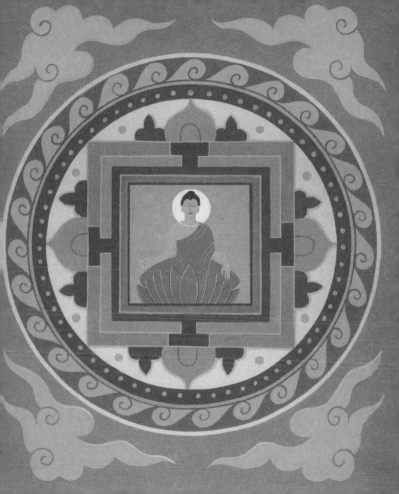

660 **Find the still point within** The world is constantly spinning. It's pointless to try and stop it. Instead, in each yoga asana, seek to find a still point – where you can relax and truly be yourself.

661 **THE STILL POINT** *"Praise and blame, gain and loss, pleasure and sorrow come and go like the wind. To be happy, rest like a great tree in the midst of them all."*
THE BUDDHA (c.563–c.483BCE), INDIA

662 **Draw energy into your core** If you draw plenty of fresh oxygen into the core of your body during asana practice, you'll feel more balanced and able to put worries in perspective. To do this, imagine drawing in energy around your navel as you hold a pose and initiate any movements from this part of the body.

663 **Ground yourself** The powerfully grounding **Eagle Pose (321)** focuses your mind and draws energy inward when you feel scattered. Fix your gaze on a chosen point and hold the pose in stillness for several seconds. This posture also gives your shoulders and arms a reassuringly deep stretch.

664 **Beginner's mind** Shed anxieties about "being good at" asanas and treat every yoga class as your first, whether you have been practising for one day, ten years or a lifetime. This allows yoga to remain creative, rather than being another pressure in your life.

665 **Finding bliss** If you practise asanas without worrying about trying to achieve perfection, you may glimpse the blissful awareness of the present moment that awaits all yogis.

666 **ONE DAY AT A TIME** *"Take therefore no thought for the morrow: for the morrow shall take thought for the things of itself."*
THE GOSPEL OF ST. MATTHEW 6.34

667 **Great calming gesture** *Maha Mudra* This practice, which helps to ease emotional pain, is useful for people under extreme stress. Sit with one leg outstretched and the other leg bent, heel to groin. Exhaling, fold forward over the outstretched leg. Keep your upper body long, tuck in your chin and don't round your spine. Reach your arms to your lower leg or, if you can manage it, to your foot. Hold for 2–3 minutes, change sides, then relax.

668 **Turning the Wheel mudra** *Dharmachakra Mudra* In this yogic gesture, your hands form wheels, symbolizing the cycle of life. Place both hands in *Jnana Mudra* **(96)**, tips of index fingers and thumbs touching. Place your right hand higher than your left, with the palm of your left and the back of your right hand facing your heart. Bring your left middle finger to touch the point where your right index finger and thumb meet (symbolizing the transition from one cycle of being to another). Ask your "higher self" to guide you through life's difficult cycles as you hold this mudra.

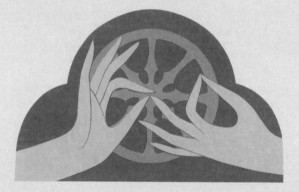

669   **Breath is the key** The sage Patanjali states that much anxiety, confusion and scattered thinking result from erratic breathing. Observe your breathing as often as you can. When it seems in any way shallow or "ragged", take a few moments to breathe deeply and slowly, in order to regather yourself.

670   **CALM BREATH, STILL MIND**
"When the breath wanders, the mind also is unsteady. But when the breath is calmed, the mind too will be still, and the yogi achieves long life. Therefore, one should learn to control the breath."
HATHA YOGA PRADIPIKA (MID-14TH CENTURY)

671   **Cooling Breath** *Sitali* This technique cools an overheated mind and body, and calms your body's systems. Slightly part your lips and curl up the sides of your tongue. Raise your head slightly and inhale your breath through your curled tongue, as if it's a drinking straw. You should hear a smooth sipping sound. At the peak of the breath, lower your chin, close your mouth and exhale through your nose. Repeat 12 times in total, if comfortable.

DEALING WITH LOSS

672 **Stop the world!** Yoga teaches that feeling exhausted by an experience is a sign that you have depleted your life-giving prana. To rebuild your energy reserves during tough times, disengage from the outside world through meditation, *dhyana* (see Sanskrit, above).

ध्यान

673 **SAVE YOURSELF** *"A wise man loses nothing, if he but save himself."*
MICHEL DE MONTAIGNE (1533–1592), FRANCE

674 **Time-out Pose** Doing a semi-inverted pose restores your body's essential systems when they are struggling from exhaustion after a traumatic experience. Lie on the floor with your legs supported on the seat of a chair, then place your palms on your lower belly, feeling it rise and fall as you breathe, until you feel rested. > 676

675 **A PLACE OF REFUGE**
"This perfect state untouched by suffering is called yoga."
BHAGAVAD GITA (400–300BCE), INDIA

676 **Supported Bridge Pose** To gently stretch the abdomen, which relieves the type of nervous tension created by emotional trauma, lie on your back with your knees bent and feet flat on the floor, hip-width apart and parallel to each other. Lift your hips and place a yoga block beneath your sacrum (the back of your pelvis) so that your pelvis is higher than your chest. Rest in this position until you feel a little more at ease, then relax. **>** 677

677 **Reclining Hero Pose** *Supta Virasana* This restorative variation of **Hero Pose (591)** helps you to surrender to the changes a loss can bring. From kneeling, widen your feet and sit between your heels (or on a yoga block). If and when you feel completely at ease in the pose, lean back, aiming for your back, head and arms to relax onto the floor (or a firm bolster). Rest here for as long as is comfortable. Then relax in **Child's Pose (864)**. **>** 683

678 **FINDING ACCEPTANCE** *"Be patient with all that is uncertain in your heart ... Do not search for answers, which will not be given: you will not be able to live them, and it is important to live everything."* RAINER MARIA RILKE (1875–1926), AUSTRIA/GERMANY

679 **Silent healing** Yoga views silence as a
deep healer. When you're suffering in the
aftermath of a loss, lie down in a quiet place,
cover yourself with a blanket and put on an eye mask.

    Seascape visualization (680) To enhance this relaxation, close
your eyes and imagine you're close to a vast ocean on a sunny
day. Inhale the sea air, holding it in your lungs for a moment
before letting it go, along with any troubling thoughts. Turn your
face to the sun and draw energy from the light. Aim to retain
awareness of any comforting sensations after opening your eyes.

681 **POWER OF SILENCE** *"True silence is the rest of the mind; it is to
the spirit what sleep is to the body, nourishment and refreshment."*
WILLIAM PENN (1644–1718), ENGLAND/USA

682 **Nerve-soothing practice** To lessen the stress that accompanies
grief, practise seated forward bends such as **Stretching the West
Pose (683),** with your chest supported by cushions. Also try
Legs-up-the-wall Pose (483). Hold the poses for longer than
usual, breathing deeply and lengthening your exhalations.

683 **Stretching the West Pose** *Paschimottanasana* This forward
bend stretches the back of the body – known as "the west" in
yoga – which stimulates *sushumna*, the primary energy channel
running along your spine, to restore energy after any emotional
loss. Sit with your legs stretching forward. Inhaling, lift your
breastbone, and exhaling, fold forward from your hips. Rest
your hands on your legs or catch your toes. Take 10 breaths,
letting go of any thoughts. Then relax. ➤ 704

684 **Supported bending** If your body feels drained or stiffened by
the stress of loss, sit on a yoga block to help you to really ease into
forward bends like **Head-to-knee Pose (480)** and **Stretching
the West Pose (683)**. Then loop an open belt around your foot
and pull the ends to lengthen your spine as you stretch forward.

685 **Ease your body** Yoga asanas not only help to "realign" your
annamaya kosha, physical body or "sheath" (see p19), and your
pranayama kosha, energetic "sheath", but also your *manamaya
kosha*, lower mind "sheath", your *vijnanamaya kosha*, wisdom
"sheath" and ultimately your *anandamaya kosha*, "bliss" body.

[265]

686 **Three Secrets Mudra** *Tse Mudra* Use this hand gesture, as Taoist monks do, to chase away sadness and help you to come to terms with loss. Kneel with your buttocks on your heels. Place your hands on your thighs, palms up, crossing the tips of your thumbs over your palms to touch the "roots" of your little fingers. Slowly inhaling through your nose, wrap all four fingers over your thumbs on both hands, making closed fists. Hold your breath while you silently say *OM* 7 times. Exhaling, unravel your fingers and draw your navel gently toward your spine. Imagine releasing all your fears and stresses with the out-breath. Repeat a minimum of 6 times, then gently stretch out your body.

687   **Notice the seasons** Since the stages of human life echo
the seasons of the natural world, spending some time
observing nature as it changes around you over the course
of a year may help you to accept the many changes and losses
that accompany growing older.

688   **NATURE'S HEALING** *"Climb the mountains and get their good
tidings. Nature's peace will flow into you as sunshine flows into trees."*
JOHN MUIR (1838–1914), SCOTLAND/USA

689   **The soul's return** The *Bhagavad Gita* tells us that death is merely
a shedding of your physical body. Your soul, as a divine and
eternal splinter, will return to the cosmic cycle: *"For certain is death
for the born, And certain is birth for the dead; Therefore over the
inevitable thou shouldst not grieve."*

690   **Think light** Whatever your loss, whether of a loved one or
of a job, try to look to future growth by repeating the following
affirmation, *"Healing light fills the void of my loss, illuminating the
way to a positive future."*

691   **ENDURANCE LESSON** *"Yoga teaches us to cure what need not be endured and endure what cannot be cured."*
B.K.S. IYENGAR (BORN 1918), INDIA

692   **Vital focus** In order to turn our convictions into reality, we must be resilient enough to bounce back from any setbacks along the way. The ability to remain focused is essential in this quest: practise **Candle Gazing (254)** to increase your focus.

693   **Mind like the restless wind** In the *Bhagavad Gita*, Arjuna, the protagonist, struggles with his restless mind. His inability to stay the course mirrors a universal human struggle. He seeks advice from his teacher, Krishna: *"O Krishna, the mind is restless, self-willed, turbulent and hard to train: to master the mind seems more difficult than to subdue the restless winds."* Krishna counsels him to build resilience through regular practice and detachment.

694   **A WORTHWHILE EFFORT** *"The harder the struggle, the more glorious the triumph. Self-realization demands very great struggle."*
SWAMI SIVANANDA (1887–1963), INDIA

695 **Stoke the inner fire** To maintain your zest for life in a hectic world, stoke the "fire in your belly" that cultivates your sense of drive, with challenging asanas such as **Boat Pose (704)**.

696 **ALCHEMY** *"All the means of action ... lie everywhere about us; what we need is the celestial fire to change the flint into crystal."* HENRY WADSWORTH LONGFELLOW (1807–1882), USA

697 **Mantra for courage** The *bija mantra*, or seed sound, *RAM* (pronounced "rum") is said to induce confidence and focus by activating the energy centre associated with the power of the sun, behind the navel – *manipura* chakra. Sit upright and repeat this mantra quietly at the end of your asana practice or when you need a sense of enhanced resilience – both physical and mental.

698 **Foods for strength** If you're coming down with a cold, reach for succulent seasonal fruit and vegetables and eat them either raw or lightly steamed. Eating them in this close-to-natural state not only ensures maximum nutrient intake but also maximum prana intake – both boost resistance to illness.

699 **A PILOT IN TRAINING** *"I am not afraid of storms for I am learning how to sail my ship."*
LOUISA MAY ALCOTT (1832–1888), USA

700 **Ride the waves** We need a stable, strong vessel to carry us over the sea of *samsara* – life's turbulent cycles. Let asanas be your boat, balancing your body, centring your mind and emotions, and cultivating the energy to ride life's storms.

701 **WAVES OF TRUTH** *"Smooth seas do not make skilful sailors."*
AFRICAN PROVERB

702 **Emotional release** To restore your zest for life when you feel worn down, practise **Camel Pose (447)**. This backbend intensely stretches the front of the body, releasing the negative emotions we store there – a cleansing that frees up space for renewed energy.

703 **DOWN AND UP** *"Our greatest glory is not in never falling, but in rising every time we fall."*
CONFUCIUS (551–479BCE), CHINA

BOAT POSE

Navasana

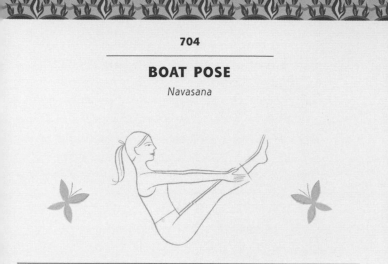

This pose strengthens the body's core, helping you to feel centred enough to bounce back after a crisis. As you do it, imagine yourself floating over problems, showing resilience to storms that can overshadow your life.

Sit on a yoga mat (with a blanket beneath it for padding). Plant your sitting bones firmly, bend your knees and hug your thighs into your belly. Without collapsing your belly or spine, lean back slightly and take your knees forward and away from you. If you can, extend your heels to straighten your legs, then stretch out your arms parallel to the floor. Hold, then relax. ❯ 737

705   **Finding a form** Different styles of hatha yoga (see pp20–23) advocate practising asanas in a different order, and with a slightly different emphasis. It doesn't matter which yoga style you choose to follow: the important thing is that you find a style that works for your own unique needs.

706   **Dig for water** If we are to move along the yoga path toward wholeness, we must, advises Krishnamacharya, settle on one style of hatha yoga (see pp20–22) and deeply explore it with a constant heart. To find water, he says, we dig a deep hole in one place, not lots of random holes like a mole disrupting a garden!

707   **EUREKA!** *"Within is the wellspring of Good; and it is always ready to bubble up, if you just dig."*
MARCUS AURELIUS (121–180), ROME

708   **Prescription for strength** To help you to deal with and bounce back from difficult situations, think about how you can cultivate *santosha* (contentment with what is) and *tapas* (disciplined practice) in both your yoga practice and your everyday life.

709 **WATER WINS** *"In the confrontation between stream and rock, the stream always wins – not through strength, but through persistence."*
THE BUDDHA (c.563–c.483BCE), INDIA

710 **Resolute mind** The *Tao te Ching* tells us that the wisest and highest warrior disarms his enemies with the power of his mind alone. Be a diplomat, aiming to resolve all conflict with persistent *ahimsa*, non-violence, like Gandhi and Nelson Mandela.

711 **WORK FOR PEACE** *"To succeed, you must have tremendous perseverance, tremendous will. Have that sort of energy, that sort of will, work hard, and you will reach the goal."*
SWAMI VIVEKANANDA (1863–1902), INDIA

712 **Keep smiling** When it feels like things aren't going your way, try to stay positive – smile! Smiling releases feel-good endorphins to help you to respond constructively in stressful situations.

713 **LOOK BEYOND THE SURFACE** *"Every tear has a smile behind it."*
IRANIAN PROVERB

714 **Resilience mudra** *Shivalinga Mudra* This hand gesture calls on the symbolic powers of the phallus of the god of change, Shiva, to fortify you to break down negativity. Make a fist with your right hand and extend your thumb upward (as if hitch-hiking!). Place this hand in the palm of your upturned left hand, which is cupped like a bowl, or mortar, with fingers together. Place your hands in front of your abdomen. Recall a negative thought or something that tries your resilience, and place it mentally in the palm of your left hand. Slowly move the pestle (your right hand) as if grinding the thought to a powder. Then blow away the imaginary dust in a gesture of dissolution.

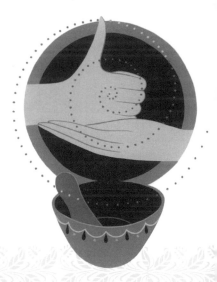

715   **You can do it** *"If you are pained by external things, it is not they that disturb you, but your own judgment of them. And it is in your power to wipe out that judgment now."*
MARCUS AURELIUS (121–180), ROME

716   **Morally resilient** To build up moral resilience, observe the five *yamas* (see p14), the foundations of yoga conduct, with awareness: *ahimsa* (non-violence), *satya* (truth), *asteya* (non-stealing), *brahmacharya* (the focused channelling of sensual energy) and *aparigraha* (non-possessiveness).

717   **Focus on success** *"The secret of success is constancy of purpose."*
BENJAMIN DISRAELI (1804–1881), ENGLAND

718   **Maintain your priorities** Consider the definition of a happy life and write down all the words that occur to you. Keep this list somewhere prominent to remind you to persist with your goals.

719   **PERSIST** *"It is never too late to become what you might have been."*
GEORGE ELIOT (1819–1880), ENGLAND

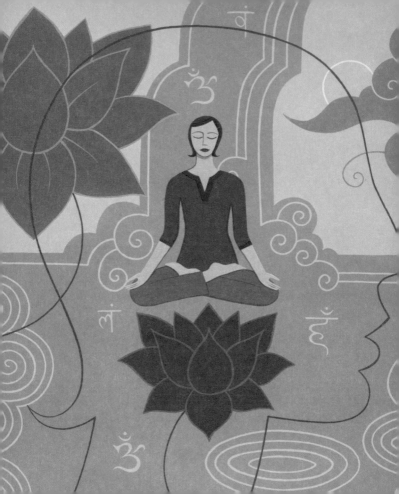

WINDING DOWN

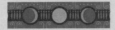

CHANGING GEAR

720   **Evening unwinding** After a busy day at work, where you've constantly had to use your brain to respond quickly and effectively to other people, reconnect with your body by showering, changing clothes and doing something to mark the transition between work and rest, such as making a cup of herbal tea or putting on some relaxing music.

721   **Respect everyday acts** The *Bhagavad Gita* urges us to treat even the most mundane daily activities – such as preparing and eating our evening meal, as a spiritual practice: *"If you regulate your eating and resting, your sleep and wakefulness – harmony in all – you will find the yoga that gives peace from pain."*

722   **Early-evening yoga** An early-evening asana practice is a particularly good way to mark the transition between work and rest. Wear garments that complement the yoga mind-set: those made from natural fibres, which stretch with your body.

723   **Where do you live?** A yoga teacher was once asked, *"Where do you live?"* Pointing to her own body, she replied, *"Here!"*

724   **INTELLIGENT BODY** Your body is often smarter than you! Follow whatever pace it's advising you to adopt during your yoga practice.

725   **Pre-asana shower** Yoga is a spiritual practice that, like prayer, should be respected by cleansing yourself with water before you begin. Bathing or showering before yoga is symbolic of cleansing the inner body. At the very least, wash your face, hands and feet before beginning an evening yoga practice.

726   **WATER'S CLEANSING POWERS**
"When you hear the splash
Of the water drops that fall
Into the stone bowl
You will feel that all the dust
Of your mind is washed away."
SEN-NO-RIKYU (1522–1591), JAPAN

727   **Clean space** Extend yogic *saucha*, cleanliness, to your yoga space at home by clearing clutter before asana sessions. This removes negative energy, which, in turn, enhances your practice.

[279]

728   Feel your throat chakra The chakra at your throat, *vishuddhi* (see p18), governs the energy with which you interact and communicate. After spending a demanding day with others, sit and contemplate its *yantra*, or visual representation (see right). Imagine the energy symbolized by its 16 vibrant petals emanating from your throat to restore you in preparation for another day's encounters.

729   Raven Beak Mudra *Kaki Mudra* This yogic gesture made with the mouth and eyes cleanses the mouth, gums and upper digestive tract. It has a cooling effect that helps you to slow down in the evening or at the end of an asana session. Sit with your spine upright, form your mouth into an "O" shape and focus your eyes on the tip of your nose. Inhale slowly through your mouth, close your mouth and hold your breath for 10 seconds, without strain. Exhale very slowly through your nose. Repeat 10 times.

730 **Tune into your own rhythm** Your energy levels move in cycles throughout the day, affecting your ability to accomplish different activities. Assess how much energy you have when you arrive home in the evening to ensure an appropriate yoga practice. For instance, if you feel tired, opt for a **Nerve-soothing practice (682)**, or if you have excess energy, try a **Playful practice (360)**.

731 **Twilight practice** For a calming evening yoga session, practise poses that bring about introspection. These include forward bends such as **Head-to-Knee Pose (480)** and **Stretching the West Pose (683)**, and inversions such as **Shoulderstand (843)**.

732 **Seated poses** Generally more contemplative than standing asanas, seated asanas, such as **Easy Pose** (p33) and **Hero Pose (591)**, have a meditative effect, so they are suitable as a winding-down evening practice. However, don't dismiss them as a physically easier option for times when your energy is low: it is more challenging to maintain an upward lift in the spine from a seated pose than from a standing one, which is why beginners usually learn to build strength and alignment in standing poses first.

733 **Go slow** What's the rush? Life is wonderful. Slow down and simply enjoy living, breathing and learning in every moment.

734 **Tune into your gearbox** Take your attention to your pelvis, imagining it as your body's gearbox – the place through which all movement passes. During an evening asana practice, try to focus on what feel like low-gear postures and movements.

735 **Shifting power** Yogis believe that by "listening" to your body's power centre, or *hara*, behind your navel, you can tune into your body's natural, or *somatic*, intelligence. Focus your attention on this area at the close of each working day and respond to what it tells you: if it suggests a need to slow down, then do so.

736 **Evening twists** Twisting poses such as **Seated Spinal Twist (737)** iron out the stresses and strains of a busy day. Your body is more flexible in the evening so it can be tempting to twist without awareness. To avoid this, first stabilize your lower back by grounding your sitting bones, then twist your thoracic spine (around your rib-cage) and finally your cervical spine (your neck).

SEATED SPINAL TWIST

Marichyasana

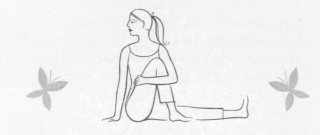

This pose is dedicated to the sage Marichi – the son of Brahma and, in Hinduism, the father of humanity. A safe, foundation-stage twist for all levels, it will help you to detach yourself from daily tribulations.

Sit with both legs outstretched, lifting your spine. Bend your right knee up and draw your right heel toward your right buttock. Maintain a hand's space between your right foot and left thigh, then hug your left arm around your right knee. Twist to the right and place your right hand behind you on the floor. Take 10–20 steady breaths, repeat to the left, then relax. ▶ 761

738 **LOOK WITHIN FOR RELAXATION** *"Tension is who you think you should be. Relaxation is who you are."*
CHINESE PROVERB

739 **Introspection** If you spend all day at a busy workplace, by the evening you may have over-worked the part of your personality that interacts with others and neglected your inner needs. This conflict between the inner and outer selves is a common theme in many spiritual traditions. To touch base with your inner self at the end of the working day, simply close your eyes and allow yourself to sit quietly for a while. Enjoy the silence and breathe deeply.

740 **WHICH BIRD ARE YOU?**
"Like two birds on the selfsame tree, the ego and the soul sit side by side in the body. The former stares about him, pecking at the sweet fruit, indulges and tastes the fruits of life, while the latter watches, discriminating."
MUNDAKA UPANISHAD (800–400BCE), INDIA

741   **Mandala meditation** A mandala is a circular pattern used
for meditation and religious devotion. To refocus your energies
at the end of a hectic day, you might like to gaze at a mandala
for 10–20 minutes (see p257). Allow your
eyes to range over its colours and patterns,
absorbing the images and motifs rather
than trying to interpret their meaning. Lose
yourself in this magic "circle" as it guides
your subconscious toward deeper peace.

742   **Turn off your mind** The spiritual teacher Eckhart Tolle estimated
that he felt most at peace when he managed to slow down his
thinking by about 80 per cent. Try to do this after a busy day by
closing your eyes and just "watching" any thoughts that arise on
an imaginary screen, without engaging with them. This shifts
your mind away from what yogis call *citta* activities (thinking,
judging, labelling etc) and from *ahamkara*, an "I"-centred focus
(in which we may spend much of our day), bringing about the
sense of peace that Tolle described. Yogis know this as *buddhi*,
a "spacious", pure and non-judgmental quality of awareness.

TIME FOR REFLECTION

743   **REFLECT ON THE WORLD** *"Regard this fleeting world like this: like stars fading and vanishing at dawn, like bubbles on a fast-moving stream, like morning dewdrops evaporating on blades of grass, like a candle flickering in a strong wind."*
THE BUDDHA (c.563–c.483BCE), INDIA

744   **Meditation class** If you find it hard to stop thinking about unresolved tasks when the time comes to stop work at the end of the day, guided meditation can help enormously. Look for a class in your local area.

745   **Sit to reflect** The Sanskrit word *dukha* means "a negative space" and *sukham* "a positive space". If you feel frazzled in the evening, sit in **Easy Pose** (p33), which takes its Sanskrit name, *Sukhasana*, from *sukham*. This pose settles an agitated body and soothes your nerves, helping to shift your mood from negative to positive.

746   **Affirm the positive** After a trying day, sit and say these words to build positivity: *"All events will flow toward a beautiful resolution."*

747   **Great Energy Lock** *Maha Bandha* Activating this empowering
"lock" – which entails harnessing three subtle "locks" in the body –
draws in energy from your extremities, and concentrates it in your
core. Learn this with a teacher first. Then, once you've learned it,
sit in **Easy Pose** (p33) and inhale deeply. Exhaling, contract your
pelvic floor to engage *Moola Bandha* **(70)**, suck your abdomen
toward your spine to practise *Uddiyana Bandha* **(114)**, then place
your chin on your chest to activate *Jalandhara Bandha*, the throat
lock. Release and relax; repeat several times if comfortable.

748   **Assimilate your day** After a non-stop day with little time
for yourself, the mindful movements of a short evening asana
practice will draw your focus away from outside demands and
help your inner light, or *prakasha*, to shine again.

749   **Hara breathing** To sense your power centre, or *hara*, which
can help to reaffirm your self-esteem after a draining day, lie
in **Corpse Pose (931)**, breathe gently and focus on your navel.
Inhaling, feel it rise; exhaling, feel it fall. Continue until you feel
your breath being drawn from deep within your *hara*.

750 **All inside** If, at the end of a busy day, you feel as if you haven't "achieved" your goals, reflect on the fact that what's inside you is enough. Union with yourself is the essence of yoga.

751 **SELF-QUEST** *"The fabled musk deer searches the whole world over for the source of the scent which comes from within."*
SRI RAMAKRISHNA PARAMAHAMSA (1836–1886), INDIA

752 **Inner-light vizualization** Yoga is a quest to connect with the divine light within, or the universal soul, however you understand it – Brahman in Hindu (see Sanskrit, right). To reflect on this, visualize light illuminating your muscles and joints as you do asanas.

ब्रह्मन्

753 **THE DIVINE IS UNIVERSAL** *"It makes no difference whether you worship God, Jehovah, Allah, Mohammed, Buddha, Christ or Krishna – it is still and always one and the same God."*
SWAMI SATYANANDA SARASWATI (BORN 1923), INDIA

754   **Sacred mantra** To take time out and reflect on your place
in the world, repeat these words from the *Katha Upanishad*:
*"May we be protected. May we be nourished. May we work together
with great energy. Let what we study be invigorating. May we not
resent each other. OM. Peace."* This Sanskrit invocation is said to
build awareness of your inner sacredness.

755   **Peace chant** If you're feeling negative, chant the final part
of the passage above in Sanskrit. *OM shanti* (pronounced "aum
shanty"), means *OM* peace. Regular chanting of this will help
to bring about a deep sense of peaceful focus and calm.

756   **Peace Mudra** *Shanti Mudra* This yogic gesture helps you to gain
a gradual sense of increased spiritual connection. Place your
hands on your navel, focusing your breathing here for a few
moments; then, take your hands to your heart, shifting the focus
of your breathing; next, move them to your forehead, focusing
your breathing here; lastly, stretch them to the sky, concentrating
on the crown of your head. Repeat, relaxing more each time you
shift your hands further up your body and further up the chakras.

757   **JUST REFLECT** *"A yogi ... lives on this earth like any other human being. He thinks, enjoys and eats like others. The great difference ... is that he has awakened a dormant faculty called ... awareness."*
SWAMI SATYANANDA SARASWATI (BORN 1923), INDIA

758   **Become a watcher** Yoga asks us to develop an observing mind, rather than getting overly caught up in life's dramas. When your mind feels tangled in the day's events, gaze at the brow-chakra *yantra* **(973)** for five minutes to connect with the "third eye" that "sees" past, present and future, and thus widens your perspective.

759   **BE AWARE** *"He [the yogi] is always aware. He is called a drashta – a seer. He is the witness of events. Your aim on the path to realizing and awakening your dormant potential should be to eventually unfold this faculty of awareness within yourself."*
SWAMI SATYANANDA SARASWATI (BORN 1923), INDIA

760   **Eyebrow Mudra** *Shambhavi Mudra* To develop a self-reflective awareness – the wisdom of the third eye – guide your gaze between your eyebrows while doing **Face of Light Pose (761)**.

FACE OF LIGHT POSE
Gomukhasana

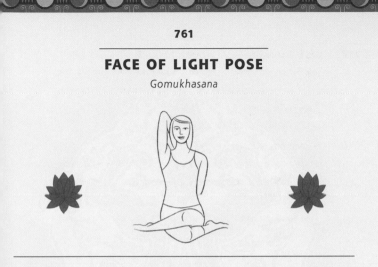

Gomukh means "cow face" in Sanskrit: some see the bent elbows and legs of this pose as the ears and lips of India's sacred animal. As it is a seated pose it encourages reflection, while stretching your spine, arms and hips.

Kneel, drop your hips to the right and cross your left leg over your right, buttocks on the floor and knees forward. Stretch your right arm over your head and bend your left arm behind your back, elbow pointing down. Then bend your upper arm and reach your hands toward each other, right palm facing in and left palm out. Hold for 5 breaths. Change sides, then relax. ▶ 782

762 **Four life stages** Vedic philosophy divides the human lifespan into four stages, or *ashramas* **(765–768)**. This word derives from the Sanskrit *shram*, meaning "work", since each stage has goals for both worldly achievement and inner development. You can use these yogic "anchors" to focus you at different stages of life.

763 **OUR INNER JOURNEY** *"Man desires objects when tender in age, enjoys them when young, seeks yoga in middle age, develops detachment when old."*
SRI TIRUMALAI KRISHNAMACHARYA (1888–1989), INDIA

764 **Reflect on the day** The stages of the day can be compared to the traditional Indian stages of life. Morning equates to the first stage **(765)**, when you carry out a lot of tasks, laying the ground for the rest of the day; afternoon to the second stage **(766)**, a time to work with deeper focus; evening resembles the third stage **(767)**, a time to unwind, withdraw from work and devote time to yourself; bedtime equates to the final stage **(768)**, a time for introspective practices such as meditation.

765 **The first stage of life** The Vedic texts recommend that in the *Brahmacharya ashrama* – the stage of "youth", from birth to age 25 – we focus on attaining knowledge, building a career and establishing material stability. The focus of your yoga practice during this phase should be asanas of all types to build a strong body that is fit for your life's journey.

766 **The second stage of life** *Grihatha ashrama*, the "householder" phase of life, from the age of 25 to 50, is a time, say the Vedic sages, to settle into a home and family life, try to fulfil our emotional needs and satisfy our ambitions. This is a time to reflect on the themes of stability and nurturing, and to settle your body by practising all types of asanas and pranayama techniques.

767 **The third stage of life** *Vanaprastha ashrama*, from the age of 50 to 75, is known as the "hermitage" phase. In India, this is considered to be the time of life when you retire from obligations, set children on their own way and pursue a spiritual life. This is a good time to reduce your asana practice and develop contemplation or meditation.

768   **The fourth stage of life** *Sannyasa ashrama*, the final phase of life, from the age of 75 to 100, is the traditional time in India to become more detached from the material world and to avoid activities in order to maintain inner equilibrium. This is the time to focus on the spiritual side of your yoga practice – *dharana* (concentration), *dhyana* (meditation, or contemplation) and *samadhi* (enlightenment).

---

769   **AWAY FROM IT ALL**
"He who wishes to withdraw should live peacefully in the forest in the third quarter of his life ..."
BHAGAVAD GITA (400–300BCE), INDIA

---

770   **Chakra reflection** Sitting for 5 minutes to contemplate a chakra (see pp16–19) can help you to come to terms with issues that come up in different areas of your life. Reflect on your **Base Chakra (59)**, **Sacral Chakra (107)** and **Navel Chakra (186)** to counter any difficulties at home, in relationships and in your work life, respectively. Reflect on your **Heart Chakra (448)** to strengthen your ability to deal with conflict in your emotional life.

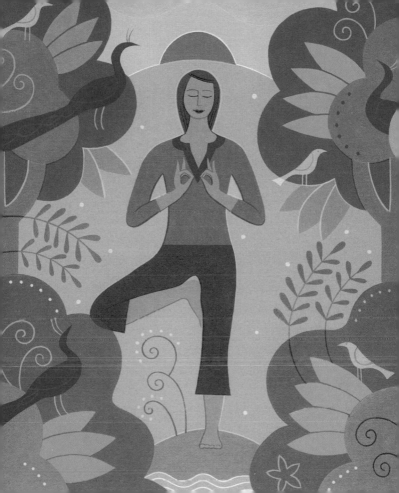

771   **DIGGING DEEP** *"Practice is cultivating inner awareness to discover depths of meditation and to realize psychological and spiritual insights into the nature of things. Practice is the active work of the individual transforming himself or herself."*
CHRISTOPHER TITMUSS (BORN 1944), ENGLAND

772   **Respect the cycle** In many ancient cultures, the first two days of the menstrual cycle were viewed as a time for women to withdraw and reflect. Today, women often do not allow for changes in both body and mind at this time, which can exacerbate stress. Aim to tune into your body and mind's need for time out and reflection.

773   **A reflective time** In the first two days of the menstrual cycle, avoid strong asana practice altogether. Use your usual yoga posture time to sit in meditation. You might try the **Full moon meditation (427)** or **Tibetan bell meditation (555)**.

774   **TOTAL SURRENDER** *"To the mind that is still, the whole universe surrenders."*
LAO TZU (c.604–c.531BCE), CHINA

775   **Life stages** Yoga wisdom teaches that women going through menopause experience less negative symptoms if they set aside daily time for reflection or meditation, which enriches you with the extra prana you need to move into a new stage of life. During these quiet times, practise the rebalancing **Alternate Nostril Breathing (69)** or the soothing **Hara breathing (749)**.

776   **Deep waters** If you find yourself avoiding contemplation or meditation because they stir up emotions you'd rather not experience, try to view inner turmoil as "growing pains" forcing you to dive within and find the resources to meet challenges.

777   **Still inside** Asanas show us that the body is never the same: from one practice session to the next, its capabilities and energy levels change. However, by closing your eyes and looking into your heart, you see that the self that lies deep inside is constant.

778   **FEELING SECURE IN YOURSELF** *"And remember, no matter where you go, there you are."*
CONFUCIUS (551–c.479BCE), CHINA

AIDING DETOX

779 **PURE BODY AND SOUL** *"The body is your temple. Keep it pure and clean for the soul to reside in."*
B.K.S. IYENGAR (BORN 1918), INDIA

780 **Travel light** To be able to travel light through life, you need to shed the emotions and thoughts that weigh you down, as well as to cleanse the body of toxins that can lead to illness. To achieve the former, explore both **Psychic cleansing (801)** and **Unblocking visualization (802)**.

781 **The energy of elimination** Yogis teach that *apana vayu*, the body's downward-moving energy of expulsion, is located in your pelvis, legs and feet, and by enhancing this energy, you detox the body. Do this with **Wind-relieving Pose (782), Wide-legged Seated Forward Bend (789)** and **Release Pose (810)**.

782 **Wind-relieving Pose** *Vatnyasana* By massaging your internal organs, this pose stimulates digestion and elimination. Lie on your back with your knees bent up and your feet flat on the floor, hip-width apart. Draw one leg toward your chest, hugging your shin as you exhale so that your front thigh massages your abdomen. Inhaling, switch legs. Repeat 10 times in total. Then relax. **>** 783

783 **Supine Twist** *Jathara Parivartanasana* Squeeze out gut toxins with this twist. Lie on your back and hug your right thigh into your belly, as in **Wind-relieving Pose (782)**. Holding your right shin with your left hand, draw your right leg across your body. Hold for 10–20 breaths. Release and change sides. Then relax. **>** 789

784 **Once a day** You should have a bowel movement at least once a day, and it should be soft and smooth in texture. If you go less often or your movements have a different texture, follow the five pillars of yogic living (see p23) to bring you into balance.

785 **Relax to let go** Stress causes the body's sympathetic nervous system to trigger a "fight-or-flight" response, diverting energy away from your internal organs to allow you to either fight or run away. This negatively affects your body's digestive and excretory functions. Asanas and meditation switch on the parasympathetic nervous system, which helps these systems to function smoothly.

786   Cleansing dynamic practice Repeating sequences of poses, or *vinyasas*, is especially cleansing for beginners. It warms the muscles, opens the energy pathways and boosts circulatory flow around the body to facilitate detoxification. Begin your practice with the Sun Salutation sequence (see pp28–31), then try **Chair Pose vinyasa (98)** and **Horse Pose vinyasa (129)**.

787   Adding to the repertoire Once you have mastered some core asanas, such as those in the Sun Salutation sequence (see pp28–31), continue to add in new poses at regular intervals. This "cleanses" the body by making your muscles and joints work in new ways and by stimulating the internal organs.

788   Cleansing forward bends Holding forward bends for longer than usual and emphasizing the exhalation aids digestion and detoxification. It also induces calm at the end of a long day, switching on the destressing parasympathetic nervous system, which aids elimination. Try the following: **Wide-legged Standing Forward Bend (204)**, **Stretching the West Pose (683)**, **Wide-legged Seated Forward Bend (789)** and **Child's Pose (864)**.

789   **Wide-legged Seated Forward Bend** *Upavistha Konasana* This pose stretches the pelvic organs by opening the hips, which promotes elimination. Sit with your legs outstretched and spine straight, then open your legs wide. Take your torso forward, bending from your hips and resting your palms on the floor between your legs. Don't curve your back in an effort to descend lower into the pose; instead keep it extended. Hold the pose for as long as feels comfortable, then gently come back up. ❯ 810

790   **PURIFYING WISDOM** *"Cleanse the fountain if you would purify the streams."*
AMOS BRONSON ALCOTT (1799–1888), USA

791   **Detox massage** Place your right hand on the lower right-hand side of your rib-cage. Your liver, here, is the primary detoxifying organ in your body, and twisting to the right massages it. As you practise the following poses to the right, then the left, imagine your liver being gently squeezed to encourage good functioning, and your body being refreshed: **Twisting Triangle Pose (357)**, **Seated Twist (619)** and **Seated Spinal Twist (737)**.

792   **HEALTHY BODY, STRONG MIND** *"To keep the body healthy is a duty ... otherwise we cannot keep our mind strong and clear."* THE BUDDHA (c.563–c.483BCE), INDIA

793   **Inner cleansing** Try a week- or month-long cleansing diet twice yearly – spring and autumn are traditional seasons in India, building your diet around fresh produce and wholefoods. (Consult a doctor if you're pregnant or have a health condition.)

794   **Rehab** Avoid additives and stimulants – caffeine, alcohol, tobacco and sugar (CATs) – to apply *ahimsa*, non-violence, to your body.

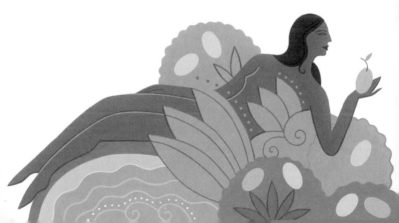

795   **Clear out your kitchen** To extend the observance of *saucha*,
cleanliness (from the second of hatha yoga's limbs, see p14), to
your home, clear your refrigerator and cupboards of out-of-date
food. Having a clearer living space detoxes your mind, too.

796   **Make your own** Cooking using fresh, seasonal ingredients,
rather than relying on pre-cooked supermarket meals, is in
keeping with the five pillars of yogic living (see p23). If you don't
know where to start, make up some simple salad dressings and
marinades for fish and vegetables by blending olive oil, garlic,
fresh herbs or spices, lemon juice and soy sauce.

797   **Use your nose** Yoga teacher Adil Palkhivala believes that
breathing through the mouth makes the heart feel "heavy" as
it prevents us from fully relaxing. To counter this, try to breathe
in and out through your nose. This filters the air and is believed
by yogis to make it more "refined", or rich in prana.

798   **BODY PARTS** *"The mouth is for eating, the nose is for breathing!"*
B.K.S. IYENGAR (BORN 1918), INDIA

799 **YOGA CONDUCT** *"Take responsibility; rid your body of its impurities; let your speech be true and sweet ..."*
SRI TIRUMALAI KRISHNAMACHARYA (1888–1989), INDIA

800 **Off your back** In **Cleansing forward bends (788)**, visualize negative thoughts and anxiety literally sliding off your back as you bend forward, leaving in their place room for positive attitudes to develop.

801 **Psychic cleansing** Sit comfortably, close your eyes and look into the dark space. Allow images and ideas to appear on this "mind-screen". Watch them without becoming involved with them for several minutes. This is known as *citta kash dharana*, mind-screen concentration, and clears the subconscious in a way similar to dreaming. If you become attached to any thoughts (by following their stories), tell yourself they are just projections on a screen.

802 **Unblocking visualization** To "detoxify" your life of anything which blocks your liberation, visualize yourself in a film, acting out a scene of your choosing in a peaceful, fulfilled state of mind.

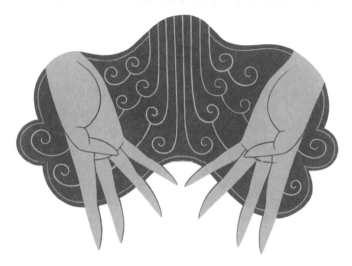

803   **Detox Mudra** This hand gesture stimulates energy circuits that
enhance the body's eliminatory organs. Place your thumbs across
your palms, pressing the tips into the root of your ring fingers.

804   **Energy-seal visualization** To relax after detoxing, visualize
brilliant light pouring from your chest to clothe you in luminosity.

ENCOURAGING RELEASE

805 ROAD TO FREEDOM *"Yoga is a way to freedom. By its constant practice, we can free ourselves from fear, anguish and loneliness."*
INDRA DEVI (1899–2002), LATVIA/INDIA

806 Primary hip release Encouraging muscular release in the body brings about a release of mental tension after a stressful day at work. Kickstart the physical release as you walk home in the evening by noticing the muscles in the back of your thighs and then the muscles in the front of your thighs. Shake out your legs as you walk to give your hips space to make their primary flexion and extension movement (forward and backward bending).

807 Limber up If you feel stiff after spending a day sitting at a desk, use the limbering exercises on pp24–26, which move the hips in six liberating directions. This also helps to raise flagging energy.

808 Evening warm-up To prepare for an evening yoga session (or ease tight legs), stand on one leg, then bend the opposite knee, drawing your thigh toward your belly. Then draw the bent leg behind you, heel touching your buttock. Repeat on the other leg.

809   **FINDING JOY IN RELEASE** *"Learn to let go. That is the key
to happiness."*
THE BUDDHA (c.563–c.483BCE), INDIA

810   **Release Pose** *Apanasana* If you feel wound-up after work or
would like to encourage release, lie on your back, bend your
knees, clasp them with your hands and hug both thighs into your
belly. Inhaling, release your thighs away from your belly slightly.
Exhaling, squeeze your thighs into your belly, as if pressing on an
accordion. This is one cycle. Repeat 9 more cycles, then relax and
feel the sensations of ease in the pelvic region. **>** 817

811   **Exhale for release** To gain more release in any asana, aim to
stretch a little further into the position each time you exhale.

812   **Easy upper body** Swinging your arms more than usual
as you walk home from work will help to limber your body
for an evening asana practice, but also frees up energy in
your heart, or *anahata*, chakra (see p18). This may be helpful
if you leave work feeling resentful or heavy-hearted.

813 **Release the shoulders** Releasing the ball and socket joint at each shoulder frees up any energy that has become "stuck" during the day. To do this, use the limbering exercises on pp24–26.

814 **Rotating palms** Awareness enhances yoga practice. Therefore, becoming aware of the key natural movements of the shoulders allows you to understand how they become tight and, to some extent, how to release them effectively. To kickstart this awareness, stretch your arms out to the sides. Turn your palms to face the sky, and feel the external rotation in each shoulder "cuff". Then turn your palms inward until they face the sky again, and feel the internal rotation. Repeat several times.

815 **Energy and space** Once you dissolve tension in your shoulders and arms and access a fuller range of motion, notice how much more energy and space you can feel in your heart and lungs: the new freedom of movement has fed them with nourishing prana.

816 **ARMS** *"… our arms extend as projections of our heart and lungs."*
DONNA FARHI (BORN 1959), NEW ZEALAND

HALF SPINAL TWIST

Ardha Matsyendrasana

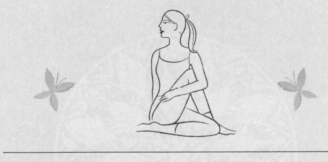

According to Hindu legend, Matsyendra, an ancient yoga teacher, performed a version of this pose for the deity, Shiva. It releases tension in the spine while balancing the left and right sides of your body.

Sit on the floor, legs outstretched. Then bend your left leg, keeping it flat on the floor, with your heel at your perineum. Lift your right leg, bending the knee, and place your right foot on the outer side of your left thigh. Twist to the right, hugging your right leg with your left hand. Enjoy the twist, keeping your spine straight, for 20 breaths. Repeat to the other side, then relax. ➤ 821

818 **IN TIME** *"Nature does not hurry, yet everything is accomplished."*
LAO TZU (c.604–c.531BCE), CHINA

819 **Breathe-easy release** Stand outside in **Horse Pose (127)** and
swing your arms, making large forward circles. Then repeat in
the other direction. Notice how this makes you breathe more
naturally and deeply, drawing fresh prana into your lungs.

820 **Heart-releasing backbends** Backbends, such as **Camel Pose
(447)** and **Passive backbend (821)**, stimulate the heart chakra
(see p18) and therefore release emotional tension. Some yogis
experience this release as a curious mix of simultaneous crying
and laughter – after which they feel emotionally lighter.

821 **Passive backbend** Sit on top of an exercise ball with both
your feet resting on the floor. Gradually ease yourself down
a little way and then slowly bend backward and lie over the ball.
Relax here for several minutes, breathing naturally. To counter the
pose, curl up in **Child's Pose (864)** on the floor, observing any
signs of physical or emotional release. **>** 842

822   **Be patient** It takes time to release into poses, such as forward bends and backbends that challenge stiff areas of your body. As you struggle to let go, ponder the words of Henry David Thoreau (1817–1862): *"Adopt the pace of nature: her secret is patience."*

823   **Spine-opening vizualisation** In backbending poses such as **Camel Pose (447)** and **Passive backbend (821)**, imagine your spine as a string of pearls, each vertebra a shining nugget threaded onto a fine silver thread of energy. Work to gently stretch the all-important cord that binds each precious pearl.

824   **NECKLACE OF SELF** *"Moderation is the silken string running through the pearl chain of all the virtues."*
THOMAS FULLER (1608–1661), ENGLAND

825   **Silk meditation** Imagine that your whole body is made of silk to encourage fluidity in your movements and therefore a sense of continuous, harmonious release. This is especially useful when you transition from pose to pose in *vinyasas*, or flowing sequences of asanas, such as the Sun Salutation (see pp28–31).

826 **Yogi Matsyendra** This ancient Indian story illustrates how yoga can free us from the pressurized constraints of modern life. When the god Shiva was teaching his wife Parvati the secrets of yoga on a riverbank, he noticed a fish eavesdropping on their conversation, fascinated by what he was saying. He sprinkled magic water on the fish, transforming him into a man so that he, too, could share yoga. Released from the water, Yogi Matsyendra (*matsya* means fish) set out to spread yoga across the globe. Think of this newfound freedom as you practise the twist named after him, *Ardha Matsyendrasana*, **Half Spinal Twist (817)**.

827 DIVINE FREEDOM *"Now the Lord is that spirit: and where the spirit of the Lord is, there is liberty."* II CORINTHIANS 3.17

828   Mantra for release OM *namo narayana* ("God is Love, Love is God") is a chant for Narayana, an aspect of Vishnu, Hindu god of maintenance, who balances everything in the universe. Chant it out loud or silently when you need to release built-up tension.

829   Wave meditation If you find it hard to wind down in the evening, sit upright, close your eyes and visualize the sea (or practise at a seashore). Watch the waves roll in and become aware of the release that comes as each wave breaks. Co-ordinate your exhalations with the breaking waves.

830   WAVE REVERIE *"Sit in reverie and watch*
The changing colour of the waves that break
Upon the idle seashore of the mind!"
HENRY WADSWORTH LONGFELLOW (1807–1882), USA

831   Peace mantra Sit and calmly sing the *bija mantra*, or seed sound, *SHAM* (pronounced "shum") to yourself in the evening. It reduces *rajas* (activity) in your body systems, ushering in deep peace.

832   **CONTENTED BODY AND MIND** *"There is nowhere to go. You are already there."*
INDIAN PROVERB

833   **Establishing your seat**
A translation of the word
asana (see Sanskrit, right) is
"to sit steady on one's own
throne". Practising asanas helps to settle you after a busy day.

आसन

834   **Lightness plus stability** To settle into a gentle evening rhythm
after a non-stop busy day, engage with three useful concepts
from the ancient yoga sages: a sense of lightness in your body,
a feeling of stability that equips you to withstand change and
a focused mind – ready for meditation.

835   **Energies of practice** Stillness and movement are polarities you
can explore in asana practice to help you to focus mindfully in an
evening session. Sense both the stillness at the core of all dynamic
movement and the movement of energy in static, still poses.

836   **A PARADOX** *"Heaviness is the root of all lightness. Serenity is the master of agitation."*
LAO TZU (c.604–c.531BCE), CHINA

837   **All through life** Asana practice is not reserved for those who are at the peak of physical condition. The renowned yoga guru Krishnamacharya said that as long as you can breathe and move your fingers, you're fit for practice. Notice how, even though your body and mind alter as you move through life, yoga allows you to feel comfortable in your skin.

838   **Restorative yoga** Relaxation poses in which your body weight is settled by being supported by "props", such as yoga blocks or a wall, suit those who are injured, stiff or exhausted. At times of diminished strength, let **Time-out pose (674)** and **Supported Corpse Pose (935)** settle tired muscles and joints.

839   **QUALITY NOT QUANTITY** *"Better is a handful with quietness, than both the hands full with travail and vexation of spirit."*
ECCLESIASTES 4.6

840   **A pose for security** When you feel vulnerable or need to
address major life issues, curl up in the protectively enveloping
Child's Pose (864) until you feel more settled. This pose is said
to recall the comforting memory of being in the womb.

841   **Chant to the Divine Mother** You might find it comforting
after a busy or unsettling day to call for support from the
nurturing energy of the universe, which in Hindu culture is
symbolized by the mother goddess Devi. Sing her mantra to
yourself: *"Jaya Jaya Devi Mata Namaha,"* meaning "I bow to the
divine mother." If you're in a group, sing the chant as a round.

842   **Shoulderstand preparation** Practising **Shoulderstand (843)**
at the end of an asana session calms you with "feminine" yin
energy. It's essential to prepare well: make a broad, firm base by
placing a folded rug, towel or four yoga blocks in a rectangular
pattern on the floor. Lie with your upper back on the raised base,
your shoulders at the edge. Let your head and neck settle slightly
lower than your shoulders on the floor. The shoulders are your
platform; don't begin the pose until comfortable. **>** 843

SHOULDERSTAND

Sarvangasana

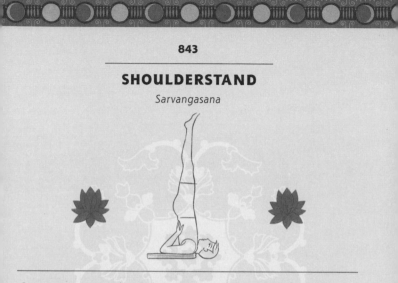

Sarvangasana means "the whole body" in Sanskrit, so it is unsurprising that this posture affects your entire being, bringing it to healing equilibrium.

Lie flat on your prepared base **(842)**. Gently bring your legs overhead, with your hands over the kidney area of your back, fingers pointing upward. Create a supportive, square platform with your upper arms (from shoulders to elbows), then aim to draw your pelvis over your shoulders. Extend your legs up and hold for 30 breaths, or as long as is comfortable. Come down from the pose in the same slow, careful way that you went up into it. Then relax. ▶ 854

844 **Settling mantra** The *bija mantra*, or seed sound, *HAM* (pronounced "hum") settles the mind as well as the body. Sing it quietly to yourself when you feel insecure or emotionally unstable.

---

845 **FINDING PEACE**
"This quietness dissolves the ... burden of all woes, for when there is stillness in your heart, wisdom will also have found its peace."
BHAGAVAD GITA (400–300BCE), INDIA

---

846 **Chakra meditation** To settle the energy in your chakra system (see pp16–18), sit upright, close your eyes and concentrate on each chakra for several seconds, repeating a particular word out loud each time. At your root chakra (around your perineum), recite the word "grounding"; at your sacral chakra (near your pubic bone), recite the word "yielding"; at your navel chakra, recite "determination"; at your heart chakra, recite "giving"; at your throat chakra, recite "purifying"; at your third-eye chakra (centre of your forehead), recite "discerning". Finally, recite "surrender" at your crown chakra (crown of your head).

847   **Turning over stones** As you practise yoga, you're likely
to encounter not only physical challenges but emotional ones,
too. To overcome these obstacles, you've got to be willing to face
them, whether they're in the form of physical tightness in certain
areas, mental resistance to the idea of certain "difficult" poses,
self-critical tendencies or extreme emotions.

---

848   **STEADY AND SERENE**
*"In the state of joy, he has found truth ... Now he
is steady, unmoved by pain or great difficulty."*
BHAGAVAD GITA (400–300BCE), INDIA

---

849   **Back to basics** Whenever your health feels unsettled,
adhere to the Sivananda philosophy of five pillars of yogic
living – right exercise, right breathing, right thinking, right
nutrition and right relaxation (see p23). Visualize yourself in
good health, meeting all life's challenges.

850   **ALIGN YOURSELF** *"May the outward and inward man be at one."*
SOCRATES (469–399BCE), GREECE

851   POSITIVE REACTIONS
"The mind becomes settled when it cultivates friendliness in the face of happiness, compassion in the face of misery, joy in the face of virtue and indifference in the face of error."
PATANJALI'S *YOGA SUTRAS* (300–200BCE), INDIA

---

852   Four goals To live a fulfilling life with integrity, say the ancient yoga sages, is to achieve four aims. The first three of these aims are: *dharma* – fulfilling your responsibilities and achieving your highest potential; *artha* – gaining the basic survival tools for life, such as food and transport, in order to be able to fulfil your *dharma*; and *kama* – fulfilling your need to experience the pleasure of sensuality. These three lead to a fourth: *moksa*, which is the bliss you experience when you connect with liberated awareness.

853   KNOWING WHAT YOU WANT *"Many men go fishing all of their lives without knowing it is not fish they are after."*
HENRY DAVID THOREAU (1817–1862), USA

FISH POSE

Matsyasana

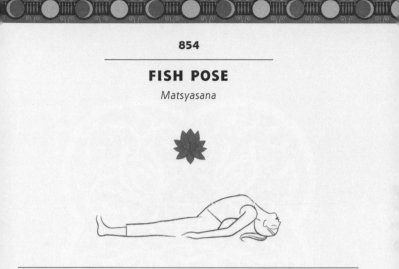

Yogic texts describe this counter-pose to **Shoulderstand (843)** as "the destroyer of diseases" because of its many health benefits. It gently extends your spine and liberates your breathing, thus settling your mind.

Sit upright with outstretched legs. Lean back on your elbows and place your hands palms down beneath your buttocks, one on each side. Pressing on the base formed by your forearms and hands, lift and open your chest to arch your upper spine., letting the crown of your head tilt back gently. Breathe in and out 10–20 times. Then lie down and relax. ➤ 864

855 **What is your dharma?** Establishing your *dharma*, your life's true course, is an important part of yoga practice. After a scattered or confusing day, it's reassuring to make a few notes that express what you believe your *dharma* to be – your responsibilities and your potential. Constantly review your notes – set aside regular time one evening a month – making changes when you see fit.

856 **TAKING CONTROL OF YOUR LIFE** *"No man is free who is not master of himself."*
EPICTETUS (55–c.135), GREECE

857 **Two pillars of a good life** To draw out your *dharma*, make sure that you observe the ethics of: *santosha* – acceptance and contentment; and *ahimsa* – non-violence. Reflect on all ten of the yamas and niyamas, the foundation observances on yoga's eightfold path (see pp14–15).

858 **Eagle Mudra** *Garuda Mudra* Making the hand gesture associated with the mythical bird Garuda, which can fly into the sun, is said to broaden your metaphorical wingspan so that you can pursue

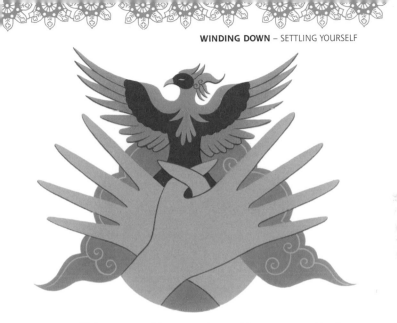

your life's purpose, with compassion and joy – unswayed by the tumult of the world. Link your right thumb over your left thumb and outstretch your hands and fingers like wings. Hold your palms in front of your lower abdomen for 10 deep breaths, then in front of your navel, next your stomach and finally your breast-bone. Feel your heart centre settle and strengthen.

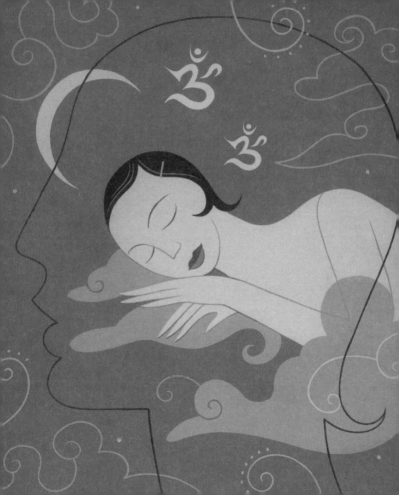

ENDING YOUR DAY WELL

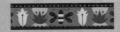

THE IMPORTANCE OF REST

859   **THE GREAT ISSUE** *"The international problem today is not hunger, poverty, drugs or fear of war. It is tension, hypertension and total tension. If you know how to free yourself from tension, you know how to solve the problems in your life. If you are able to balance your tensions, you can control your emotions, anger and passions."*
SWAMI SATYANANDA SARASWATI (BORN 1923), INDIA

860   **Physical tension** Yogic philosophy outlines three types of tension that a mindful yoga practice can help to resolve. The first is muscular tension (see **871** and **879** for the others). To sleep without tension, practise **Yoga Nidra (939–944)** before bed.

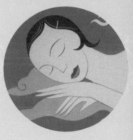

861   **Seek release** If your busy schedule has made you physically stressed, you'll benefit from the supported shoulderstand **Legs-up-the-wall Pose (483)**. Resting here for several minutes at the end of the day encourages your parasympathetic nervous system to switch on, which destresses you ready for a good night's sleep.

862 **Turn upside down** After a hectic day, invert your body to ease any strain on your heart by doing **Time-out Pose (674)** or **Shoulderstand (843)**, after preparatory limbers (pp24–7).

863 **DON'T BE AFRAID TO STOP** *"He does not seem to me to be a free man who does not sometimes do nothing."*
CICERO (c.106–43BCE), ROME

864 **Child's Pose** *Balasana* Go into this nurturing, restful pose between asanas during a gentle yoga practice or any time you need to rest. Kneel with knees together and buttocks on the heels. Fold forward to rest your chest on your thighs and your forehead on the floor. Let your arms lie by your sides, and hands by your feet, palms up. Relax, breathing deeply. ➤ 916

865 **Pranic rest** Spend 10 minutes before you go to bed in nurturing **Child's Pose (864)**, to give your body's systems time to slow down and bring about a sense of restful equilibrium.

   See your prana (866) While in **Child's Pose**, imagine your prana infiltrating all the cells of your body.

867 **Nada yoga** The word *mantra* means "sacred sound" (see Sanskrit, right), and *nada yoga*, the "yoga of sound", uses mantras to dissolve physical tension and encourage peaceful sleep. Feel the calming effects of *nada yoga* by reciting a mantra such as **Bedtime mantra (870)**.

868 **RESTFUL INNER MUSIC** *"Nada is found within. It is a music without strings which plays in the body. It penetrates the inner and outer and leads you away from illusion."*
KABIR (1440–1518), INDIA

869 **Bathe in sound** A *nada yoga* (sound-yoga) practice, such as **Bedtime mantra (870)** or **Bee Breath (928)**, prepares you well for sleep, as its sounds are thought to attune your "inner ear" to what yogis call "the subtle sounds" of restful meditation.

870 **Bedtime mantra** To envelop yourself in calm, quietly repeat to yourself the nerve-soothing *bija mantra*, or seed sound, *SOM* (pronounced "sohm"), until your body feels heavy with relaxation.

871   **Release emotional tension** As well as releasing muscular tension **(860)**, yoga recognizes the importance of releasing emotional tension arising from life's many "dualities", such as love and hate, and wealth and poverty. Yogis teach that being constantly bombarded by examples of such extremes by the media can leave you unable to properly rest, even during sleep.

872   **Turn off the TV** Following a yogic lifestyle means making evenings a time of rest rather than of stimulation and heightened emotions. Try swapping your evening TV sessions for peaceful music, a meditation or an asana practice now and again.

873   **Collective tension** If you've had any kind of altercation during the day, be sure to release any emotional tension when the evening comes. Otherwise, it can radiate out to affect your family, friends and colleagues, causing them, too, to become tense. This sets up a vicious circle of negative emotions, physical tension and even aggression that inevitably rebounds to affect you. Stop the vicious circle by releasing your emotional tension with **Legs-up-the-wall Pose (483)** or **Nada yoga (867)** before you go to bed.

874 **Let tension go** If you feel emotionally over-wrought, your abdominal region is likely to tighten up. Practise slow, rhythmic **Hara breathing (749)** to soothe this vulnerable part of your body.

875 **Rest your eyes** When thoughts spiral out of control as a result of anger or frustration, fix your eyes on a still point for respite: **Candle Gazing (254)** brings about a restful *drishti*, gaze point.

876 **A SOFT GAZE** *"When the mind relaxes, the gaze becomes drishti."*
SRI K. PATTABHI JOIS (BORN 1915), INDIA

877 **One focus** If you rest your gaze on a point with **Candle Gazing (254)**, your mind is drawn into *eka-grata*: one-pointed awareness. This is an important step toward *dharana*, concentration, yoga's sixth limb (see p15) and the door to meditation.

878 **What is yogic concentration?** *"Dharana is holding the mind within a centre of spiritual consciousness in the body, or fixing it on some divine form, either within the body or outside it."*
PATANJALI'S *YOGA SUTRAS* (300–200BCE), INDIA

879   **Cause of mental tension** Yogis recognize that mental tension arises when myriad thoughts of past or future experiences whirl around in your mind – all clamouring for attention at once. They call this state of mind *citta*.

    Whirlpool visualization (880) To calm a mind racing with too many thoughts, imagine a heron sitting by a swirling pool of water. Watch how he disregards the surface commotion, only delving into the pool to pluck out life-sustaining fish when the moment is absolutely right – to avoid wasting any energy. Try to emulate this focus when it comes to your own scattered thoughts.

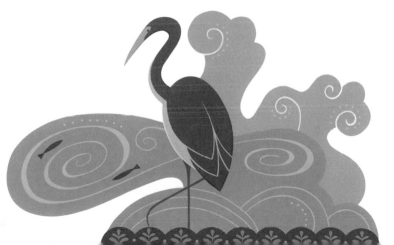

881 **YOUR PLACE IN THE WORLD** *"Accept the place the divine providence has found for you, the society of your contemporaries, the connection of events."*
RALPH WALDO EMERSON (1803–1882), USA

882 **Current-of-peace meditation** Sit upright, close your eyes and visualize a smooth-flowing river. View the flowing water as a gentle current of peace. Launch yourself into this nurturing current. Feel immersed in, and comforted by, its fluidity and gentle strength; and let it draw you toward a vast, silent lake, where it feels easy and natural to drift into contented sleep, without anxious thoughts dominating your mind.

883 **Layers of rest** Having a sense of being at peace after using mind-calming techniques such as **Current-of-peace meditation (882)** is evidence that you're cleansing your *manamaya kosha*, the mental and emotional "sheath" of the body (see p19).

884 **Uncover your higher self** Using the practical techniques in this chapter helps you to experience greater physical and mental rest, which vitalizes your *vijnanamaya kosha*, the intelligence sheath linked to dreams, intuition and higher awareness (see p19). This is rather like pruning an overgrown garden, clearing unwanted growth to allow something truly beautiful to grow.

885   WEEDING THE MIND *"Our bodies are our gardens, to which our wills are gardeners."*

WILLIAM SHAKESPEARE (1564–1616), *OTHELLO*, ENGLAND

886   Retire from the material world One of the key messages of the ancient yogis is that focusing on the material side of life alone cannot make us truly happy, as we are always likely to want "more". Make a conscious decision to give yourself a break from unnecessary material consumption. After a few weeks, notice whether you feel more at rest within yourself in bed at night.

887   REMOVE DESIRES *"When one withdraws all desires as a tortoise withdraws its limbs, then the natural splendour of the world soon manifests itself."*

MAHABHARATA (c.400BCE–c.200CE), INDIA

888 **Rest your brain** Most of us allow the part of the brain that governs logic to rule our day. But relying too heavily on this aspect of our mind prevents us from finding inner peace because it chokes the mind with calculation, projection, judgments and prejudice. After a hard day, give your brain some down time by tapping into your intuition and acting spontaneously.

889 **End the day creatively** Try to take 20–30 minutes in the evening to pursue a creative activity, such as writing or drawing. This uses the part of your brain associated with inspiration and intuition, thus ending the day on a gentle, self-nurturing note.

890 **Develop your intuition** It is a good idea to schedule a regular evening meditation "slot", as valuable and intuitive thoughts often emerge during such sessions. Rather than overthinking these, just write them down and come back to them the next day.

891   **ACCESS A DEEPER KNOWING** *"You must hear the birds' song
without attempting to render it into nouns and verbs."*
RALPH WALDO EMERSON (1803–1882), USA

892   **Intuition mantra** Repeating the *bija mantra*, or seed sound, of
the third-eye chakra, *OM* (pronounced "aum"), opens your mind to
intuition, resting the conscious brain. While you say it, imagine the
clouds in your mind clearing, as you sink into a restful blue sky.

893   **Koan meditation** Zen meditation uses short phrases called
koans to disrupt the linear-thinking mind that always searches for
logical solutions. Before bed, rest your logic by pondering the
koan, *"Show me your face before your mother and father met."*

894   **Bedtime request** Say a prayer at bedtime for the deep rest
that comes when you trust in a greater being.

895   **THE PEACE OF TRUTH** *"The soul enjoys silence and peace,
not by many reasonings, but by simply contemplating the Truth."*
ST PETER OF ALCANTARA (1499–1562), SPAIN

MINDFUL RELAXATION

896 **What is relaxation?** Most people assume that relaxation is what happens when you lie down. Try instead to think of relaxation as yogis do – as a state free from muscular, emotional and mental tension. This may take time to achieve, depending on how much tension you have accumulated over the years, but all the practical pearls in this book will help you on your journey toward it.

897 **HEAVENLY RELAXATION** *"Unite closely your mind and body. Can you stay focused on their perfect harmony? In regulating your breath to attain softness, can you reach the state of a newborn child? You will see heaven in every direction if you are able to cleanse your inner vision."*
LAO TZU (c.604–c.531BCE), CHINA

898 **Dissolving yourself** To become truly relaxed, it's important to work toward dissolving your sense of separate identity (which yogis know as *ahamkara*), replace it with a sense of being connected with the universe (a state of mind known as *buddhi*).

   Relaxation in motion (899) Think about the following example of the sense of oneness described above: In order for a Zen artist to do his work, he must embody relaxation. To paint a stalk of bamboo, he must therefore firstly concentrate upon the bamboo until he loses consciousness of himself and becomes at one with the bamboo. Then when he paints, he does so with the rhythm and the spirit of the bamboo.

900   **RESOLVING DIFFERENCE** *"... oneness is the secret of everything."*
SWAMI VIVEKANANDA (1863–1902), INDIA

901   **The seventh limb** When your attention no longer vacillates, you experience *dhyana*, or meditation, the seventh of yoga's eight limbs (see p15). Patanjali explains, "Dhyana *is the unbroken flow of thought toward the object of concentration."*

902   **Body, breath and mind** In Patanjali's eight-limbed yoga path (see pp14–15), we are urged first to practise physical poses, which give the body the flexibility to sit quietly and comfortably; next, to work on breath-control exercises, which cleanse the energy channels, allowing prana to flow freely; and then to do meditations, which calm the busy mind. For ultimate relaxation, structure home sessions around this successful formula.

903   **The bliss of relaxation** Yoga texts describe the awareness of
your *anandamaya kosha*, or bliss sheath (see p19), the innermost
layer of consciousness, as a condition of total relaxation and
"bliss". You become aware of this body by permeating the four
outer layers of consciousness during meditation, especially
through the guided relaxation of **Yoga Nidra (939–944)**.

904   **Seed-sound meditation** "Re-tuning" the chakras by chanting
their seed sounds settles your energy when you feel uptight
and can't physically or mentally relax enough to wind down
before bed. Sit upright and take your attention to each chakra
in ascending order, sounding out its *bija mantra*, or seed sound.
Start with the base chakra in your perineum, chant its sound *LAM*
(pronounced "lum"). At your sacral chakra, around your sacrum,
chant *VAM* ("vum"), at your navel chakra sing *RAM* ("rum"), at your
heart chakra *YAM* ("yum"), at your throat chakra *HAM* ("hum")
and at your third-eye and crown centres chant *OM* ("aum").

905   **REPAIR WORK** *"In stillness the world is restored."*
LAO TZU (c.604–c.531BCE), CHINA

906 **Undo inner knots** Breathing is to the mind what asana is to the body: a tool to unravel inner knots that stop you from relaxing. Use it to counter problems such as ingrained negative attitudes and sheer mental exhaustion to help to put you in a peaceful state of mind before sleep. Pranayama exercises like **Lengthening the out-breath (907)** help to remove any mental and emotional blockages that build up, making you feel more at ease within.

907	**Lengthening the out-breath** To induce a tranquil mind, watch the flow of your breath through your body. Notice how this diverts your mind from other distractions. Then, gradually lengthen each out-breath, or *recaka* (see Sanskrit, below), until it becomes twice the duration of the inhalation, or *puraka*. After a few minutes, notice how much more relaxed you feel.

रेचक

908	**Sitting for meditation** The best sitting pose for meditation, **Thunderbolt Pose** (see p33) makes you feel relaxed and tuned into your inner world, yet simultaneously alert. It is used for prayer by Japanese Buddhists and forms part of the *salaat* (prayer) sequence of Muslims. If at first you find it hard to relax your feet or legs in the pose, place a yoga block or firmly folded blanket beneath your sitting bones, but if you have knee problems, opt for **Gracious Pose (916)** instead.

909	**Yoga stillness** Once you have settled into a sitting pose such as **Thunderbolt Pose** (see p33) or **Gracious Pose (916)**, try to sense the dynamic nature of your stillness. Aim for your body to be completely relaxed; your breath to feel serene; and your mind to remain fully aware. This is true relaxation, so don't worry if you only catch glimpses of it.

910 **AT ONE** *"No thought, no action, no movement, total stillness: only thus can one manifest the true nature and law of things from within and unconsciously, and at last become one with heaven and earth."*
LAO TZU (c.604–c.531BCE), CHINA

911 **A little, often** If you find sitting in stillness brings physical or mental stress rather than relaxation, try not to give up. Practise little and often – a much more effective strategy than an occasional blitz of intensity. Remember the Chinese aphorism that the journey of a thousand miles begins with a single step ...

912 **EXPAND YOUR HORIZONS**
"O Krishna, the stillness ... which you describe is beyond my comprehension."
BHAGAVAD GITA (400–300BCE), INDIA

913   **Subtle energy centres** Induce a yogic feeling of relaxed well-being before bed by devoting some time to rebalancing your body's chakras, or subtle energy centres.

Chakra rainbow meditation (914) To achieve a sense of this balanced well-being before sleep, sit upright and close your eyes. Focus on the base chakra and visualize a ball of red energy glowing there. Moving upward, concentrate on the sacral chakra and see a glowing orange ball. Next, picture a yellow ball at the navel chakra. Then, focus on the heart chakra where you see a glowing green ball. Next, concentrate on the throat chakra and see a light blue ball. Higher still, visualize an indigo ball at the brow chakra. Lastly, focus on the crown of your head, where a violet ball shines. Finally, visualize all the chakras glowing at the same time, before gently "closing" each chakra by revisiting it and shrinking its energy to a point of light. Then relax.

915   **Whole and relaxed** By attuning yourself to your internal life-force with chakra meditations **(846)** and **(914)**, you become aware of layers of consciousness beyond the physical body (see p19). This makes you feel more whole and so more relaxed.

GRACIOUS POSE

Bhadrasana

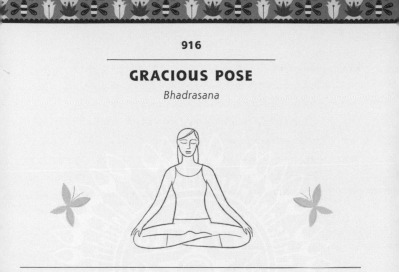

This pose is sometimes called "the posture of the throne", as its grounded, triangular base supports a noble, yet comfortable, seated position. It is an easier yet just as effective alternative to **Thunderbolt Pose** (p33).

Sit on the floor with your spine upright and your legs open wide. Draw one of your feet in, resting the heel beside your perineum. Draw in the other foot and balance it on top of the first foot.

Rest your hands on your knees, palms downward. Once you feel comfortable here, you can practise any meditation in this position. Or, you can simply rest in this pose. ➤ 931

917 **Heart focus** To still heightened emotions or develop compassion during evening relaxation, sit, close your eyes, and, when your mind and body feel still, use your "inner eye" to look at your heart. Just hold your focus here for as long as feels comfortable.

918 **Fan the flame** Contemplative techniques such as **Metta Meditation (457)** and **Heart focus (917)** are thought to fan the "eternal flame", or divine spark, which is said by the ancient yogic texts to lie in a cave at the back of your heart. Practise these techniques in order to recognize and connect with the divine element that is inherent in everything in life.

919 **Restoring relationships** Having the ability to truly relax makes both your social and home life feel more whole, because it gives you not only the ability to switch off from work but also the energy to connect with family and friends in a more heartfelt way.

920 **A calm that cannot be swayed** *"Tranquillity is a certain quality of mind, which no condition or fortune can either exalt or depress."* SENECA (c.4BCE–65CE), GREECE

921   THE ATTRACTION OF STILLNESS

"The secret of the receptive
Must be sought in stillness;
Within stillness there remains
The potential for action."

SUN BU'ER (c.1119–1182), CHINA

922   Final relaxation Having bathed yourself in relaxation
during an evening yoga practice, end by sitting upright to
scan your body for any areas of persistent tightness – sit on
a yoga block, if necessary, to effortlessly lift your spine toward
the sky. Root your pelvis well, sending equal weight through
both sitting bones. Once you're comfortable, bring your focus
to your breath. Imagine each inhalation as a tiny stream of
light coursing through your body to illuminate any spaces
inside you that still feel tight or unrelaxed.

923   Evening affirmation To seal in the relaxing energy brought
about by an evening yoga practice, say, "I trust that the universe
will support me when I relax and follow my intuition."

[345]

DRIFTING TOWARD SLEEP

924 **Soften your mind** If you're still having trouble "switching off" once actually lying in bed, focus on your breathing by following **Lengthening the out-breath (907)**. This establishes strong connections between your body and mind which help to unravel deeply held tension and soothe your nerves, thus encouraging you to feel relaxed enough to fall asleep.

925 **SMOOTH YOUR BROW AND YOUR PILLOW** *"A ruffled mind makes a restless pillow."*
CHARLOTTE BRONTË (1816–1855), ENGLAND

926 **Bathe in sound** Use a *nada yoga* (sound-yoga) practice, such as **Bedtime mantra (870)** or **Bee Breath (928)**, as you lie in bed if you find it tricky to drift off to sleep naturally.

927 **Sheep-counting mantra** If you wake up in the night and find it hard to get back to sleep, repeat the *bija mantra*, or seed sound, *SHAM* (pronounced "shum") over and over, instead of counting sheep. After a while, this should raise you above your controlling mind – into the deep peace of total rest.

928   **Bee Breath** *Brahmari* This breathing exercise is named for the sleepily hypnotic humming sound that it creates inside your head. Sit with your spine straight and press your index fingers into your ears to seal off your "outer" hearing. Close your mouth, separating your teeth and relaxing your jaw. Breathe in slowly through your nose. As you exhale – again through your nose – make a smooth, continuous humming sound. Repeat several times, allowing the sound vibrating inside your head to lull you.

929   **Prana Vidya** To tap into healing energy before you fall asleep: sit upright and rest your hands in your lap, palms curved together like a cup as in **Cupping the Void Mudra (112)**. Close your eyes and breathe calmly. Inhaling, raise your hands up through the midline of your body and stretch them above your head in a gesture of openness and receptivity. Hold the inhalation for a few moments, as if drawing in prana from the ether. Exhaling, return your hands to your lap in the cup mudra. Repeat 5 times in total.

930   **SLEEP BENEFITS** *"Sleep that knits up the ravelled sleeve of care ..."* WILLIAM SHAKESPEARE, (1564–1616), *MACBETH*, ENGLAND

931 **Corpse Pose** *Savasana* This is yoga's quintessential relaxation pose, and it gives your body, mind and emotions a chance to settle and come together. Use this pose or its variation, called **Supported Corpse Pose (935)**, to end every asana session. Lie on your back with your legs far enough apart that your lower back feels at ease, feet dropping outward. Let your arms relax away from your sides, palms facing upward. Close your eyes and position your head so that you look straight up at the ceiling. Rest here for 10 minutes or longer. ❯ 935

932 **Bed breathing** Once you're lying comfortably in bed, turn your attention inward, following the thread of each breath as it leads to the next. This gives the breath and mind the space to settle into a natural, and soothing, flow.

933 **Navel focus** Lying relaxed, feel how your belly rises with each inhalation and falls on each exhalation. Count 10 breaths in and out, visualizing them as waves on a gentle ocean.

   Ajapa mantra (934) This sound of your breath in and out is *soham*, an "unspoken mantra" that induces deep tranquillity.

SUPPORTED CORPSE POSE

Salamba savasana

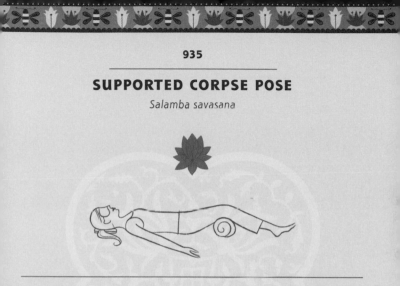

Salamba means "with support" in Sanskrit, so if you find **Corpse Pose (931)** uncomfortable, or if you feel particularly exhausted, try this variation which uses props to help your body relax into a state of profound calm.

Lie on your back with your legs apart and feet dropping outward, and a rolled yoga mat or blanket under your knees to allow your lower back to release. Place a yoga block or folded blanket beneath your head to maintain length through the back of your neck. Put on an eye mask, cover your body with a blanket and, if you wish, put on relaxing music or a yoga nidra CD. ➤ 945

936   **Deepest sleep** Electrical impulses emitted by the brain show that profound states of meditation can replicate the deepest form of sleep, with all its benefits for health and well-being. During normal waking, when rational thinking and sensory stimulation predominate, the brain emits high-frequency beta waves. In mild states of meditation, when the rational mind and senses are inoperative, the brain emits lower-frequency alpha waves. During sleep, when the unconscious predominates, even lower-frequency theta waves are emitted, associated with intense creativity. But the lowest, delta, waves – linked to receptivity and learning – come about only in deep, dreamless sleep, high states of meditation and *samadhi*, the eighth limb of yoga (see p15).

937   **Sleep-inducing mantra** To bring on very deep sleep, recite the following mantra very slowly and deliberately: *"OM HRAM, OM HRIM, OM HRUM, OM HRAIM, OM HRAUM, OM HRAM."*

938   **What is yogic sleep?** Developed by Swami Satyananda Saraswati, **Yoga Nidra (939–944)**, also known as "yogic sleep", induces such deep, systemic relaxation that one hour's practice is said to give the benefits of four hours' actual sleep. It involves the fifth limb of yoga, *pratyahara*, or withdrawal of the senses (see p15).

939 **Yoga Nidra** Prepare by lying in **Corpse Pose (931)** in a quiet, warm place. Remain still but alert as you follow pearls **940–944** (have someone read them to you or record them to play back).

Start Yoga Nidra (940) As you lie still, become aware of every part of your body, from the crown of your head to the tip of your toes. Mentally say the mantra *OM* and then recite a short *sankalpa*, or positive resolve, such as, "I am vibrantly healthy."

Gradual relaxation (941) Direct your relaxed focus to your right thumb for a moment, followed in turn by each finger, then the palm and back of your hand, your wrist, lower arm, elbow, upper arm, shoulder and armpit. Then turn your attention to relaxing your hip, thigh, kneecap, calf, ankle and heel; the sole of your foot, top of your foot, and each toe in turn. Repeat this gradual process of relaxation on the left side of your body.

Relaxation continued (942) Next, become aware of the back of your body: your right and left shoulder blades, right and left buttocks, your spine and entire back. Then focus on your front: the crown of your head, your forehead and temples, your right and left eyebrows, the space between your eyebrows, your right and left eyes, your right and left ears, your right and left cheeks, your nose, mouth, chin, throat, each side of your chest, your abdomen and your navel. Focus on your right leg, your left leg, both legs; your right arm, your left arm, both arms. Then, focus on your whole back, your whole front and your whole body.

Breathing and visualization (943) Next, notice how your navel rises and falls with your breathing – rising as you breathe in and falling as you breathe out. Then, in order to awaken your creative eye, fix your attention on each of the following images for a few seconds before switching to the next: a burning candle, an endless desert, a rushing stream, a red mountain, a temple at dawn, birds flying across a sunset, stars at midnight, a white lily, and gentle waves in the eternal sea.

End Yoga Nidra (944) Finally, repeat the resolve **(940)** 3 times, with conviction. Then release all effort and repeat *OM* silently before returning your awareness to your body. Gently stretch, and then roll onto your side to rest before getting up.

YOGIC SEAL

Yoga Mudrasana

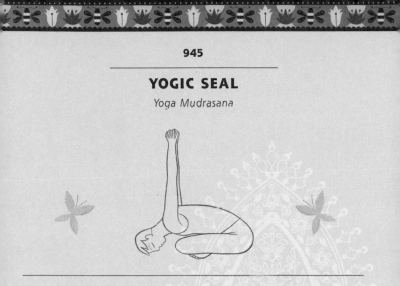

This "seal" posture forms the traditional conclusion to asana practice, so folding into it is an excellent way to round off a series of poses. Allow it to "seal off" the day you have just had and mark the transition to night-time.

Sit on the floor cross-legged and clasp your hands together behind your back. Inhaling deeply, lift your chest and look up. Exhaling, fold forward and take your brow as close to the ground as you can, raising your arms behind you toward the sky. Relax here as you take 10 smooth breaths. Gently return to the sitting position and observe your breath before relaxing in **Corpse Pose (931)**.

TRANSFORMATION

946   **Lucid dreaming** Yoga transforms our inner world by developing powers of visualization and imagination, and heightening intuition. Practise **Yoga Nidra (939–944)**, an especially powerful exercise in inner transformation, to enter a state between wakefulness and sleep in which the mind becomes especially alert and open to positive auto-suggestion.

947   **WAKEFUL DREAMING** *"The psyche of man is dreaming all the time, consciously as well as unconsciously. The dreams we have at night are only a small part of this totality."*
SWAMI SATYANANDA SARASWATI (BORN 1923), INDIA

948   **Transform your life** Yoga prescribes meditation for clearing the subconscious of longstanding behavioural habits that hold us back. Once you have established a regular meditation practice, you'll be more able to control your thoughts and also to allow your dreams to inform your waking choices.

949   **CHOICE OF ROLES** *"In the world of dreams, I have chosen my part."*
ALGERNON CHARLES SWINBURNE (1837–1909), ENGLAND

950   **A wider world** A Chinese folk tale tells of a frog who lived inside a well, so content with his life within it that he could not contemplate leaving it. One day, his cousin appeared, exclaiming, "Where I live is vast; there are no walls." "Not possible!" replied the frog. But eventually, he visited his cousin, who lived near the ocean. The frog was speechless to find that, indeed, this huge expanse of water had no boundaries, and when he opened his eyes, which were used to darkness, he saw that it was flooded with a dazzling, mind-blowing light. Having seen the wonder of the wide world outside his well, he never returned home again. When you fall asleep, try to leave your mind open to this ocean of light and to possibilities you have not yet experienced.

951   **Connection with the elements** Both the physical world and the spiritual body are composed of five elements, known as the *panchabhuta* in Sanskrit – earth, water, fire, air and ether. Finding a connection with these elements through meditation as shown in **Element meditations (952–957)** can help us to deepen our understanding of our composition, and heighten our sense of being made of the stuff of nature.

[355]

952   **Element meditations** During your evening meditation, let your mind absorb the unique qualities of each of the elements as well as of the five chakra centres in order to become more aware of your energetic and spiritual aspects.

Earth (953) Close your eyes and contemplate the element earth: think about its grounding qualities and focus on your base chakra. Imagine the earth dissolving in water.

Water (954) Next, think about the qualities of pure flowing water: consider its fluidity and clarity before taking your focus to your coccyx (where your sacral chakra is located). Imagine a pool of water vaporized by a great heat.

Fire (955) Now think about the transformative power of fire, and focus behind your bellybutton (your navel chakra). Imagine the tip of the flame dissolving into the air around it.

Air (956) Turn your thoughts to the light, spacious qualities of air, then focus on the area of your chest behind your heart (your heart chakra). Draw a few deep breaths into your heart.

Ether (957) Finally, think about invisible, all-expansive ether and focus on your throat chakra. Imagine light-infused space bathing your body before gently opening your eyes.

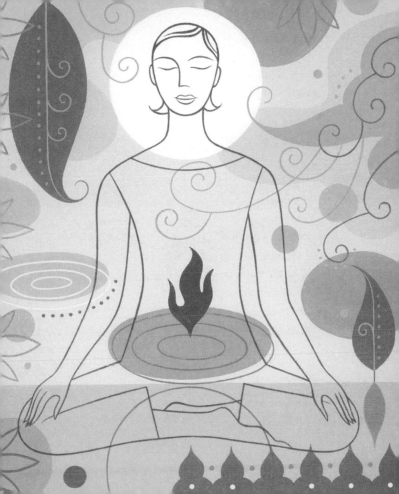

958 **From matter to spirit** The awakening of spiritual consciousness is a gradual, quiet process. Don't look for spectacular signs or *siddhis* (spiritual powers and gifts): this distracts from the path.

959 **THE CONCEALED PATH**
"The path of grace does not reveal itself to one who blunders through the world totally committed to it and its limitations. It is a subtle hidden path never revealed to one who thinks that this world is all there is ..."
KATHA UPANISHAD (800–400BCE), INDIA

960 **Quiet, but steadfast** In the *Yoga Sutras*, Patanjali warns us to stay awake – on the lookout for transformation – at all times. He explains: *"Distraction due to past impressions may arise if the mind relaxes its discrimination, even a little."*

961 **AN EVER-MOVING PATH** *"But be aware: remain ever vigilant, for even this state of yoga can ebb and flow."*
KATHA UPANISHAD (800–400BCE), INDIA

962   **A blissful state** When your mind is clear, pure and untainted
by judgments, you see things as they really are – you have
reached *samadhi*, the eighth limb of yoga, or an equal and
balanced way of thinking (see p15). You might catch an
occasional glimpse of this blissful state when practising
one of the meditations in this book.

963   **RECOGNIZING REALITY** *"When in meditation, the true nature
of an object shines forth, not distorted by the mind of the perceiver,
that is absorption (samadhi)."*
PATANJALI'S YOGA SUTRAS (300–200BCE), INDIA

964   **OM mantra** The yogic texts state that reciting the sound
of **The creation mantra (8)** – *OM* (pronounced "aum") –
is transformative, as it unites you with everything that is. Sit
upright, take a deep breath in and, as you exhale with an
open mouth, allow each of the three sounds of the chant *OM* –
"aaa", "uuu" and "mmm" – to emerge in turn. Feel them resonate
within your whole being. Then inhale and repeat the chant again
on the next exhalation, to create a continuous flow.

965 STREAM OF CONSCIOUSNESS

"Like the continuous flow of an oil stream and like the vibration of a bell. This is the way to pronounce OM and the way to really know the meaning of the Vedas."

DHYANABINDU UPANISHAD (800–400BCE), INDIA

---

966 Exploring OM When you feel comfortable chanting *OM* **(964)**, speed up your repetition, keeping your awareness on the individual sounds, or synchronize your chant with the rhythm of your heartbeat to become really at one with it. Then take the *OM* chant inward by repeating it silently, yet still imagining the sound resonating in every cell of your body.

---

967 THE POTENCY OF OM

"OM is the unsurpassed means for taking you from the glorious Self within to knowledge of the Self beyond. Contemplation of Om will lead you into that blissful realm of the ultimate reality."

KATHA UPANISHAD (800–400BCE), INDIA

968 **Meditating on OM** Breaking down the Sanskrit character *OM* (see right) into its consituent parts (in terms of both visuals and meaning) shows you the journey this mantra leads you on – into the subtle, spiritual realms.

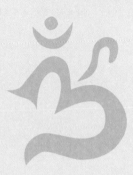

Find your conscious mind (969) Look at the top curve of the "3" shape. This is *"aaa"*, signifying your conscious, waking mind.

Drop to your subconscious (970) View the lower loop of the "3" shape. This is the sound *"uuu"*, which denotes and taps into your subconscious, a far greater space than the waking mind.

Discover your unconscious (971) Find the separate curved line flowing out from the junction of the main "3" shape – this is the sound *"mmm"* and relates to your unconscious. Then find the little half-moon above the main symbol – this is *maya*, the veil of illusion that masks the deep truth of transcendental awareness *turiya*, which is represented by the dot, or *bindu*.

972   BEYOND TIME

*"The mantra OM is the universe. It is Brahman
(the absolute). It is time – past, present and future.
It is also that which transcends time."*

MANDUKYA UPANISHAD (800–400BCE), INDIA

---

973   Feel your brow chakra The subtlest of the chakras is *ajna* (see
p18), situated at the central point between your eyebrows. It is
considered to be a "third eye", or eye of intuition, which looks
inward rather than outward when functioning well, and governs
your extra-sensory perception. To develop this chakra, gaze at its
simple but beautiful *yantra*,
or visual representation (see
right). Alternatively, simply
close your eyes and for
several minutes try to
sense the location of this
pure and subtle centre
behind your eyes in the
seat of your brain.

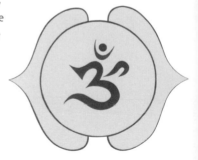

974   **ALL-SEEING SOUL** *"... in every man there is an eye of the soul, which ... is more precious far than ten thousand bodily eyes, for by it alone is truth seen."*
PLATO (c.429–c.347BCE), GREECE

975   **Power point** A lesser-known energy centre, called the *bindu*, lies at the back of the head, behind your brow chakra **(973)**. This is the subtle centre from which the human psychic framework is said to arise and is where the finite world we know connects with the infinite world of which yoga makes us aware. The Sanskrit word *bindu* means a "dot" or "point", and implies a dimensionless energy centre with the infinite potential of the number zero.

976   **Transforming mind** Don't struggle to understand your *bindu* **(975)** with your rational mind – it can't be approached in this way. You begin to perceive it only through yoga practices.

977   **POTENTIAL OF ZERO** *"On the yogic path, the mind has to become like a bindu – infinitesimally concentrated yet with unlimited potential."*
SWAMI SATYANANDA SARASWATI (BORN 1923), INDIA

978 **LET GO** *"Let yourself be worn out; you will be renewed. Once you have let go of your desires, you will receive everything."*

LAO TZU (c.604–c.531BCE), CHINA

979 **Life in death** As you sink into **Corpse Pose (931)** at the end of an asana practice, think about its Sanskrit name *Savasana* (*sava* means "corpse"). Devout yogis welcome this metaphorical death as a freeing experience, a shedding of the mortal coil that keeps us earthbound. Think of each *Savasana* as a symbolic death that offers you the chance to release aspects of yourself that you wish to shed, and to metamorphose into a new skin.

980 **STUDY FOR THE SOUL** *"Life is the soul's nursery – its training place for the destinies of eternity."*

WILLIAM MAKEPEACE THACKERAY (1811–1863), INDIA/ENGLAND

981 **A last exhalation** We tend not to exhale enough during the day, focusing instead on inhalations, which can leave us very tense. In the last moments of the day, let go with **Lengthening the out-breath (907)** or **Exhalation breathing (982)**.

982   **Exhalation breathing** Make each exhalation before bed profoundly deep. As you exhale, imagine releasing any remaining physical tension; let everything go. Notice how when you exhale more deeply you feel more at peace: the ego is breathed out.

983   **FEEL FEAR** *"... we are so afraid of life itself that we have not known it, we have not entered deep into it. That creates the fear of death."*
OSHO (1931–1990), INDIA

984   **The final release** By emphasizing exhalation as we wind down for sleep, we show a willingness to let go of the day and we acknowledge that only by resting can we be re-invigorated to live fully tomorrow. Similarly, yogis contemplate death as a natural part of life's flow and a way of asserting just how alive we are now. Thinking about death forces you to let go of the fears that stop you from really living, and allows you to embrace life.

985   **OPEN UP** *"Death is the transformation of the envelope that contains our spirit. Do not confuse the envelope with its contents."*
LEO TOLSTOY (1828–1910), RUSSIA

SILENCE AND SURRENDER

986   **THE QUIET PATH** *"It has often occurred to me that a seeker after truth has to be silent."*

MAHATMA GANDHI (1869–1948), INDIA

987   **Silence reveals all** In silence, say the Vedas, everything is revealed. If you spend time in silence, a practice known in yoga as *mouna*, you effortlessly begin to reconnect with the true self that lies deep inside you – with whom many of us have lost touch. This practice also helps you to conserve pranic energy, which makes you feel peaceful in preparation for bedtime. Try to spend at least a short period of time each evening being silent. It is particularly useful to sit or lie silently for 5–10 minutes just before going to bed.

988   **PURE, STILL SILENCE**
"Remember always – not with my speech, not with my eyes, not even with my mind will that Self be reached. It will declare itself to me only in my stillness."
KATHA UPANISHAD (800–400BCE), INDIA

989   **Inner-source mudra** *Yoni Mudra* By closing the portals of your face to the outside world, this gesture induces a wonderful silence and a palpable sense of surrender. Sit comfortably, breathing slowly. As you breathe in, seal your ears with your thumbs, press your eyelids closed with your index fingers and close your nostrils with your middle fingers. Then place your ring and little fingers over your lips to close them. Hold the inhalation without straining, then remove your middle fingers to exhale through your nostrils. Inhale again, close your nostrils and hold. Lift the fingers to exhale. If you feel comfortable, repeat several times. (Avoid if you're prone to depression.)

990   **Silent surrender** As you practise any form of silent meditation, try to surrender everything that attaches you to the world, from material desires to emotions such as anger and anxiety. Then, simply try to concentrate on the purity of the silence.

991   **FILLING THE SILENCE** *"Silence is like an upright empty glass that is capable of being filled with, and retaining, the water of knowledge."*
MATA AMRITANANDAMAYI (BORN 1953), INDIA

992   IN SILENCE, MEET YOURSELF
"Once the Self is known, that Self which sees with eyes open or shut, all sorrows end."
KATHA UPANISHAD (800–400BCE), INDIA

---

993   Well meditation If you're not sure how to explore your "inner self", lie on your back, close your eyes and visualize a deep, silent well with a bucket hanging from the top. Imagine that your mind is in the bucket, and that your breath is the rope. Slowly – over several minutes – lower your mind (in the bucket) deeper into the well by lengthening your breath (the rope). As you spend time in the cool, dark silence, in the knowledge that you can emerge any time you wish, sense your mind becoming calmer and more spacious. After a few minutes, gradually draw yourself back to the surface. Then stretch, open your eyes and feel how your renewed sense of spaciousness leaves you prepared for a deep, calm sleep.

994   REACHING A PURE PLACE *"Out beyond ideas of right-doing and wrong-doing, there is a field. I'll meet you there."*
JALAL AL-DIN RUMI (1207–1273), PERSIA

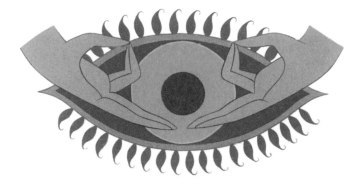

995 **Mudra for clear vision** *Prana Mudra* This is said to foster a quiet clarity of mind that helps you to rediscover your true self at the end of your day. Sit upright, place the tips of your thumbs, ring and little fingers together, stretching out your index and middle fingers. Hold, breathing steadily, then repeat several times.

996 **AWAKENING YOUR TRUE VISION** *"Your vision will become clear when you look into your heart."*
CARL JUNG (1875–1961), SWITZERLAND

997 **The crown chakra** At the crown of your head lies the highest chakra, *sahasrara* (see p18), your entry point to the spiritual world. It is depicted as a lotus with a thousand petals (see right), which symbolize the chakra's unlimited nature. It is described as *shoonya*, or "voidless void", a paradox that describes how impossible it is for us to understand it with the conscious mind, or to truly know the joy and sense of connection it can bring. Swami Satyananda Saraswati says it *"transcends all concepts yet is the source of all concepts. It is the merging of consciousness and prana."*

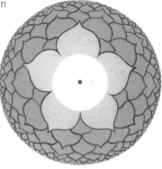

998 **Sensing the crown chakra** When all the chakras spin in harmony, a much experienced yogi may perceive the crown chakra, and, with it, the transformative, divine light of all the chakras shining in the spinal column like a string of pearls.

999 **Let go of all you know** To be able to get in touch with the *bindu* **(975)** and crown chakra **(997)**, you need a guide that is sensitive to these subtle centres. One such guide is the mantra *OM (pronounced "aum")*. At night, just before you go to sleep, try to forget everything you know and simply repeat this over and over again as you lie with your eyes closed. Surrender to it and, in the words of the great yogi Tilopa, allow it to let you "look into the mirror of the mind" and become conscious of heaven in the midst of life. Allow this yogic sound to carry you into deep sleep.

1000 **THE SECRET WITHIN THE SOUND**
"This single, imperishable sound will lead you where you wish to go. Whether you wish to know the Self, as it is embodied in flesh, or the Self as it transcends embodiment, OM will lead you there."
KATHA UPANISHAD (800–400BCE), INDIA

1001 **A final word** *"By practising Yoga, impurities dwindle away and the light of wisdom dawns."*
PATANJALI'S YOGA SUTRAS (300–200BCE), INDIA

GLOSSARY

Ahimsa: non-violence; one of the five *yamas*

Ajna: sixth or third-eye chakra, sited at the centre of the forehead, between the eyebrows

Anahata: fourth or heart chakra, sited around the centre of the chest

Antar mouna: inner silence

Anuloma Viloma: Alternate Nostril Breathing; pranayama technique

Apana: vital air, or subtle energy, of the lower abdomen

Apanasana: Release, or elimination, Pose

Aparigraha: non-covetousness or non-grasping; one of the five *yamas*

Ardha Chandrasana: Half-moon Pose

Ardha Matsyendrasana: Seated Half-Spinal Twist Pose, named after the yogi Matsyendra

Ardho Mukha Svanasana: Downward Dog Pose

Asana: pose or posture; the third limb of Patanjali's eight-limbed path of yoga

Asteya: non-stealing; one of the five *yamas*

Baddha Konasana: Butterfly, or bound angle, Pose

Bakasana: Crane Pose

Balasana: Child's Pose

Bandha: energy lock, or gate, employed to direct prana, or seal energy within the body; applied where there is an arched bone construction: at the neck, abdominal cavity, pelvic floor and feet

Bhakti yoga: the yogic path of devotion

Bharadvajasana: Seated Twist Pose, named after the Vedic sage Bharadvaja

Bhastrika: Bellows Breath; pranayama technique

Bhramari: Bee Breath; pranayama technique

Bidalasana: Cat Pose

Bija mantra: seed sound; the main six are: *LAM, VAM, RAM, YAM, HAM* and *OM*

Bindu: a subtle energy centre sited toward the back of the head

Brahma: the Hindu creator god

Brahmacharya: moderation; celibacy; one of the five *yamas*

Buddhi: pure state of being

Chakra: a subtle energy centre sited along the spine

Citta: mind-stuff; memories, thoughts and opinions

Citta kash: the cave of the mind

Dharana: concentration; the sixth limb of Patanjali's eight-limbed path of yoga

Dharma: virtue, or true way of life

Dhyana: meditation; the seventh limb of Patanjali's eight-limbed path of yoga

Dosha: qualities that make up an individual's constitution; there are three: *vata, pitta, kapha*

Ganesh: Hindu god of beginnings and remover of obstacles

Gomukhasana: Face of Light, or Cowface, Pose

Guna: quality or energy force; there are three: *rajas*, *sattwa* and *tamas*

Ida: the left, or lunar, *nadi*, or energy channel

Ishwara pranidhana: living with a constant awareness of God; one of the five *niyamas*

Jalandhara Bandha: subtle chin lock

Janu Sirsasana: Head-to-knee Pose

Jathara Parivartanasana: Supine Twist

Jnana yoga: the yogic path of knowledge

Kapalbhati: Skull-shining Breathing; pranayama technique

Kapha: earth; one of the three *doshas*

Karma yoga: the yogic path of service

Kriya: practices to cleanse the body

Kumbhaka: Suspended Breath; pranayama technique

Kundalini: latent energy sited at the base of the spine; often depicted as a coiled snake

Maha Bandha: great energy lock

Maha Mudra: great calming gesture

Mandala: symbolic, circular diagram used in meditation

Manipura: third or solar-plexus chakra, sited around the navel

Mantra: sacred sound

Marichyasana: Seated Spinal Twist Pose, named after the sage Marichi

Matsyasana: Fish Pose

Metta: loving-kindness, Buddhist form of meditation

Mooladhara: first or root chakra, sited around the perineum

Mudra: symbolic gesture of the hands, eyes or body

Moola Bandha: root, or supportive, energy lock, at the perineum

Nada yoga: the yoga of sound

Nadi: subtle energy channel through which prana flows

Nataraja: name of the Hindu god Shiva in his aspect as Lord of the Dance

Natarajasana: Dancer Pose

Navasana: Boat Pose

Niyamas: five behavioural precepts; the second limb of Patanjali's eight-limbed path of yoga

OM (or **AUM**): the most powerful sacred sound syllable; the source of all other mantras

Pada Bandha: foot, or grounding, energy lock

Padottanasana: Wide-legged Standing Forward Bend Pose

Parivrtta Trikonasana: Twisting, or revolved, Triangle Pose

Paschimottanasana: Stretching the West, or back of the body, Pose

Patanjali: author of the *Yoga Sutras* – the earliest systematic teachings on yoga

perineum: area of the body between the anus and the vulva or scrotum

Pingala: the right, or solar, *nadi*, or energy channel

Pitta: fire; one of the three *doshas*

Prana: subtle energy, or vital air

Pranayama: mastery of the breath; the fourth limb of Patanjali's eight-limbed path of yoga

Pratyahara: withdrawal of the senses; the fifth limb of Patanjali's eight-limbed path of yoga

Purvottanasana: Stretching the East, or front of the body, Pose

Rajas: quality of activity; action; drive

Sahasrara: seventh or crown chakra, sited at the crown of the head

Samadhi: highest state of consciousness; the eighth and final limb of Patanjali's eight-limbed path of yoga

Samskaras: karmic imprints, or ways of thinking that define behaviour

Sankalpa: affirmation in the present tense; positive resolve

Santosha: contentment; one of the five *niyamas*

Sarvangasana: Shoulderstand Pose

Sattwa: quality of vital balance present in all things

Satya: truthfulness; one of the five *yamas*

Saucha: purity or cleanliness; one of the five *niyamas*

Savasana: Corpse Pose

Simhasana: Lion Pose

Sitali: Cooling, or sipping, Breath

Sitting bones: the two "knobbly" bones that extend out from the base of the pelvis (at the buttocks)

Sukhasana: Easy Pose; comfortable seated pose

Supta: reclining

Sushumna: central *nadi*, or energy channel, through which *kundalini* rises

Swadhisthana: second or sacral chakra, sited around the tail-bone

Swadhaya: studying the sacred texts; one of the five *niyamas*

Tadasana: Mountain Pose

Tamas: quality of inertia; lethargy; inaction

Tantra: to weave, stretch or expand (the mind) beyond physical limitations

Tapas: austerity; one of the five *niyamas*

Third eye: point in the middle of the forehead, where cosmic consciousness develops

Tratak: Candle Gazing; a concentration technique

Trikonasana: Triangle Pose

Uddiyana Bandha: abdominal, or lightness, energy lock

Ujjayi: Victorious, or uplifting, Breath; breathing with narrowed glottis

Upavistha Konasana: Wide-legged Seated Forward Bend pose

Ustrasana: Camel Pose

Utkatasana: Fierce or Intense Pose; also known as Chair Pose

Uttanasana: Intense Pose; standing forward bend

Vajrasana: Thunderbolt Pose

Vatnyasana: Wind-relieving Pose

Vata: wind or air; one of the three *doshas*

Vedas: sacred scriptures

Vinyasa: moving sequence of asanas linked together with breathing

Viparita Karani: Legs-up-the-wall Pose

Virabhadrasana: Warrior Pose

Virasana: Hero Pose

Vishnu: the name of divinity in its maintaining, sustaining aspect in Hinduism

Vishuddhi: fifth or throat chakra, sited around the throat

Vrksasana: Tree Pose

Yamas: five ethical practices or restraints; the first limb of Patanjali's eight-limbed path of yoga

Yantra: a geometric symbol to aid contemplation; a visual depiction of a chakra

Yoga: spiritual practice originating in India; literally means "to yoke together" or "unite"

Yoga Nidra: yogic sleep; meditative technique

MENU OF KEY YOGA PRACTICES

The key yoga practices suggested in this book are grouped below, according to pearl number, to allow you to focus on any particular practical element of yoga that appeals to you at any given time. The references run sequentially through the chapters.

ASANAS
27, 45, 46, 57, 98, 99, 117, 127, 128, 129, 156, 173, 178, 204, 227, 235, 250, 283, 302, 321, 337, 357, 386, 415, 447, 480, 481, 483, 506, 534, 549, 591, 592, 677, 683, 704, 737, 761, 782, 783, 789, 810, 817, 821, 842, 843, 854, 864, 916, 931, 935, 945

BANDHAS
55, 70, 114, 747

CHAKRAS
58, 105, 186, 258, 363, 369, 448, 548, 579, 728, 846, 973, 997, 998

MANTRAS
8, 59, 90, 106, 107, 126, 187, 198, 290, 305, 324, 372, 388, 397, 465, 601, 605, 612, 646, 648, 697, 754, 828, 831, 841, 844, 870, 891, 904, 927, 937, 964, 999

MEDITATIONS
60, 85, 110, 284, 303, 393, 427, 454, 457, 515, 530, 537, 548, 555, 585, 633, 741, 825, 829, 882, 893, 904, 914, 929, 951, 961, 973, 993

MUDRAS
29, 96, 112, 135, 206, 273, 296, 328, 366, 398, 428, 455, 524, 545, 546, 611, 656, 667, 668, 686, 714, 729, 756, 760, 803, 858, 989, 995

PRANAYAMA TECHNIQUES
69, 122, 185, 212, 350, 353, 390, 463, 527, 671, 749, 907, 928

VISUALIZATIONS
14, 50, 71, 100, 109, 188, 220, 238, 298, 327, 449, 511, 522, 535, 544, 552, 575, 583, 642, 680, 752, 801, 802, 804, 823, 825, 880

375

INDEX

Note: All references in the index are page numbers (not pearl numbers, as given on page 375).

376

379

ABOUT THE AUTHOR

Liz Lark is an experienced yoga teacher, author, artist and retreat leader. Her yoga clients have included high-profile actors, dancers and many others, including The Monteverdi Choir led by Sir John Eliot Gardiner. She has authored eight books, and has created a DVD entitled *Yogalibre: A Creative Practice of Hatha Yoga* (2008). To contact Liz, or for further information about her work, yoga workshops and retreats, please visit her website: www.lizlark.com.

AUTHOR ACKNOWLEDGMENTS

A heartfelt thank you to Kelly Thompson, commissioning editor, for bringing this book to life. Thanks also to the artist, designer and editors for their inspiring and creative contributions.

PUBLISHER'S ACKNOWLEDGMENTS

The publishers wish to thank Jo Micklem and Duncan Carson for their invaluable editorial help with this project. The publishers also wish to thank those listed on p384 for their kind permission to reproduce the copyright material in this book. Every effort has been made to trace copyright holders, but if anyone has been omitted we apologize, and will, if informed, make corrections in any future edition. The publishers would also like to thank the following for their help with translation from foreign texts: Patricia Leitch, Verona Patel, Mahala Semple.